HEALTH CARE IN TRANSITION

CAREGIVERS

PRACTICES, CHALLENGES AND EXPECTATIONS

HEALTH CARE IN TRANSITION

Additional books in this series can be found on Nova's website under the Series tab.

Additional e-books in this series can be found on Nova's website under the e-book tab.

HEALTH CARE IN TRANSITION

CAREGIVERS

PRACTICES, CHALLENGES AND EXPECTATIONS

ADRIENNE LLOYD
EDITOR

nova publishers
New York

Library of Congress Cataloging-in-Publication Data

Library of Congress Control Number: 2015953171

ISBN: 978-1-63483-909-9

Published by Nova Science Publishers, Inc. † New York

CONTENTS

PREFACE

Family caregivers play a crucial role in providing daily assistance to individuals who are unable to care for themselves. Being a family caregiver can create family caregiver burden, which is discussed in the first chapter of this book. It provides a systematic review of the interventions available for family caregivers. Chapter two and three focus on quality of life and caregiver burden among caregivers of chronic liver disease patients, and epileptic patients. Chapter four examines parents' perceptions of caring for children with learning disabilities, and their psychosocial well-being. Chapter five aims to improve the understanding on disclosure trends, impacts, and factors that may inhibit or motivate children to disclose sexual abuse experiences to their caregivers. Chapter six explores the author's experiences with caregivers of children in HIV-affected Southern African communities. The final chapter studies the accuracy of health information resources on the internet that many caregivers rely on.

Chapter 1 – Background: Family caregivers play an important role to take care their loved one at hospitals or at home. There are significant differences of health status and work status between before and after being caregivers. There are many interventions that help family caregivers to relief their family caregiver burden, improve their quality of life, and psychological well-being. Few studies did a systematic review of literature of the interventions for family caregivers. Purpose: The purpose of this study was to provide a integrative literature review of interventions for family caregivers in order to provide an evidence based information for future nursing interventions. Methods: This was an integrative review research design. The peer-reviewed journal articles were searched from the following databases: Academic Search Complete, Academic Search Premier, CINAHL, MEDLINE, and PsycINFO. The key words were Intervention and Family Caregiver. The period of years of the journal articles was during 2006-2015. Results: Twenty-two research-based articles met the including criteria and were included in the review. There were 14 interventional research design articles and 8 descriptive correlational research design articles recruited. There were four categories of diagnosis in this review: (I) Heart Failure (n = 3), Coronary bypass surgery (n = 1); (II) Mental Illness (n = 1), Schizophrenia and mood disorders (n = 2), Suicide (n = 1), Dementia (n = 2), Seizure (n = 1); (III) Chronic Illnesses (n = 1), Stroke (n = 3), Incapable older people and home-care services (n = 1), Diabetes (n = 1); (IV) Cancer (n = 7), Leukemia (n = 1). There were 9 countries' studies included in this review. They were Taiwan (n = 4), Canada (n = 2), Iran (n = 5), Australia (n = 1), Netherlands (n = 1), Iceland (n = 1), United States America (USA) (n = 6), German (n = 1), and United Kingdom (UK) (n = 1). Twelve (85.71%) interventional studies had significant differences in reducing caregiver burden between pre and post test studies including Etemadifar et al. (2014), Navidian et al. (2010), Sigalet et al. (2014), Moieni et al. (2014), Sun et al. (2014), Pfeiffer et al. (2014), Northouse et al. (2013), MacNeil and Jaggers (2013), Sharif, Shaygan, and Mani (2012), Kolbrun Svavarsdottir and Olafia Sigurdardottir (2013), Pahlavanzade, Khosravi, and Moeini (2014), and Ridge et al. (2014). Conclusion:This review highlights that interventional studies have positive effects on decreasing family caregiver's burden. The factors influencing family caregiver's burden are also described. The detail interventions of these effective randomized clinical trials (RCT) are included in this review for future studies.

Chapter 2 – Chronic liver disease (CLD) and cirrhosis are currently the 12th leading cause of death in the United States [1]. Due to ongoing cost-containment efforts, there is an increased need for family-based care of chronically ill individuals. Debilitating symptoms of fatigue, pruritus, ascites, malnutrition, and encephalopathy are common manifestations of patients with CLD. The presence of CLD at home has a significant impact on the primary caregivers and affects their overall quality of life. Several studies demonstrated a significantly lower mental health component on the quality of life assessment among caregivers of CLD patients. However, only a minority of caregivers reported a formal clinical diagnosis for depression or anxiety, underscoring the fact that a significant number of caregivers may have undiagnosed clinical depression. Chronic depression and stress in the presence of inadequate resources and increasing patient dependency has been linked to decline in both physical and mental health status of patients and caregivers. While physicians are coached to "treat the whole patient," the future of longitudinal care for chronic diseases, including advanced liver disease, may require treating the person seated next to the patient as well.

Chapter 3 – The burden of caring for the epileptics places a toll on stakeholders of epilepsy management. It is hence very essential to understand the cross cultural psychology of epilepsy, origin of epilepsy, prevalence of epilepsy worldwide and the Nigerian perspective on epilepsy pathology and management of epileptics' self esteem. Epilepsy is not yet clearly understood and there is no known cure. Because of this, and the historical context, fear of the disorder is widespread. At one time the disorder was thought to be caused by the possession of a person by the devil and even today, myths, misunderstandings and social stigma still exist. As a result, the patient may fear rejection by peers and employers and decidedly refuse to disclose the health problem even though it would be wiser to do so. The epilepsies are characterized by sudden seizure caused by a disruption of activity in the brain cells. While in some cases the cause of epilepsy can be determined (usually a head injury or brain tumor), generally the origin of the seizure is unknown. It is notable that upping the self esteem of the epileptics should be paramount in psychotherapeutic management of epilepsy.

Chapter 4 – Caring for a child with learning difficulties can be both a rewarding and a difficult experience; however, little is known about parents' perceptions of caring for these children and their psychosocial well-being. This exploratory, qualitative study was conducted to explore these couples' perceived health needs in care-giving to a child with different learning difficulties (LD). A purposive sample of 22 couples who were caring for a child with LD at home were recruited from two regional child mental health centers in Hong Kong. Data were collected from individual couples with semi-structured interviews between April and June 20134. Each interview was audio-taped and lasted more than one hour. These interview data were transcribed to Chinese and analyzed by using content analysis. Four categories of parents' perceived health needs were identified, including needs for specific knowledge (and skills) about care provision, health issues of self and LD child, showing much demands for psychosocial support, and barriers to seeking helps and support. Specific health needs related to knowledge of the illness and its care, social support from spouse and health professionals, and reluctance to seek help from people were perceived as important by the parents. These results reveal important issues and challenges in providing illness- and culture-specific nursing care for these family carers. The findings can facilitate health professionals understand parental needs with regard to knowledge of the illness, psychosocial support, expectations to their child, and attitude and behavior towards help-seeking in LD caregiving. Health care providers should provide appropriate education for these families in terms of their psychosocial and culture-specific needs, in order to improve their health and well-being.

Chapter 5 – Over recent years, the number of reported cases of sexual abuse in children has increased with new and bizarre cases every day, most especially in Nigeria. However, the true prevalence is difficult to ascertain because it is a crime that flourishes in secrecy. This is promoted by the unrelenting perpetrator as well as victims' family members who wish to maintain and protect the family dignity and honour to avoid stigmatization. Disclosure is a delicate and sensitive process which is influenced by several factors, including implicit or explicit pressure for secrecy, feelings of guilt, shame, fear of negative consequences and/or embarrassment. Although, sexual abuse of children provokes reactions of indignation and incomprehensibility in all cultures, the perception and attitudes of caregivers could affect reporting of sexual abuse, prosecution of perpetrators, and provision of clinical services. The nature and quality of support and protection from caregivers provides an effective platform for quick recovery and improvement in mental health and social functioning of victims. Unfortunately, not all caregivers are supportive of survivors; instead, disclosure of childhood sexual abuse is often met with disbelief, anger, or rejection which leaves victim feeling isolated and unworthy. This paper therefore, aims at improving the understanding on disclosure trends, impacts, and factors that may inhibit or motivate children to disclose sexual abuse experience(s).

Chapter 6 – This chapter recounts the author's experiences and discusses empirical findings deriving from her research work with caregivers of children, since 2006, in HIV-affected Southern African communities. The author's entry into these caregivers' world commenced with multi-country qualitative research in South Africa and Malawi, aimed at better understanding and defining vulnerability in Southern Africa. What she observed and learned through her contact with households and communities would lead her to spend over five years conducting mixed methods research to explore the potential protective role of (family and community) social support for caregiver and child health. This chapter aims to combine the scientific with the experiential, to tell a story of challenges and resilience, despair and hope: a story that unravels over time through insights provided by both anecdotal and empirical information, as well as the author's own observations, questions and reflections. It concludes with suggested foci for future health and social support research and interventions with caregivers and children in Southern Africa.

Chapter 7 – *Introduction:* The internet is perceived as a prominent source of health information by parents worldwide. A survey study showed that 43% of the parents used the internet as a source of health information in the previous six months. More and more people are connecting with each other through social media (Facebook, Twitter, Freelyshout, and many others) and websites like PatientsLikeMe for being informed and supported, although informally. *The Physician's Role:* The physician should be ready to face requests on reliable websites and books on general or specific health issues. In a study, 67% of patients in a community-based primary care practice agreed that clinicians should be able to recommend specific websites where they could find health information. *Health Information Media:* Health information is available in print (magazines, books, newsletters) or electronic (radio, television, websites, hotlines) media. Choosing the most convenient ones will be at the caregiver"s discretion. In any case, she/he should be informed that the information is not necessarily reliable when it becomes visible to the public. *The Problem of Finding Trustworthy Information on the Internet:* According to a paper by Eysenbach et al., 55 studies concluded that quality of health information was a problem on the web, 17 studies remained neutral, and seven studies came to a positive conclusion. Positive studies scored significantly lower in search ($P = 0.02$) and evaluation ($P = 0.04$) methods. In a study by Soot et al., one third of the presented information was classified by the authors as misleading or unconventional. The authors have chosen Google, which is the most widely used search engine, to simulate a parent's experience in trying to find an answer on whether to have her/his child vaccinated against influenza. The authors searched the internet for an answer to the question "Should I make my child vaccinated against influenza?" Their findings call for the urgent need to check public-oriented healthcare information on the internet for accuracy, completeness, and consistency. *Differentiating High and Low-Quality Websites:* Studies reveal that parents' inclination to believe the correctness of medical internet information and not to discuss it with the child's physician is considerably high. Taking into account this scientifically established indispensability of internet in the eyes of the modern society, it may be more prudent to increase the quality of health information on the internet, rather than trying to dissuade people from resorting to the World Wide Web for health information or decisions. Groups, such as the OMNI Advisory Group for Evaluation Criteria (omni.ac.uk) and the Collaboration for Critical Appraisal of Information on the Net (www.medcertain.org), are refining technical mechanisms by which users of the internet can easily locate quality health information in a transparent manner based on evaluative meta-information labeling and indexing. Accreditation of websites by independent certification systems, such as HONcode, may be another solution to the quality problem of the health-related websites.

In: Caregivers
Editor: Adrienne Lloyd

ISBN: 978-1-63483-909-9

Chapter 1

Systematic Review of the Interventions for Family Caregivers

Pi-Ming Yeh**, RN, PhD,
Associate Professor, Department of Nursing and Allied Health,
Missouri Western State University, US

Abstract

Background: Family caregivers play an important role to take care their loved one at hospitals or at home. There are significant differences of health status and work status between before and after being caregivers. There are many interventions that help family caregivers to relief their family caregiver burden, improve their quality of life, and psychological well-being. Few studies did a systematic review of literature of the interventions for family caregivers.

Purpose: The purpose of this study was to provide a integrative literature review of interventions for family caregivers in order to provide an evidence based information for future nursing interventions.

Methods: This was an integrative review research design. The peer-reviewed journal articles were searched from the following databases: Academic Search Complete, Academic Search Premier, CINAHL, MEDLINE, and PsycINFO. The key words were Intervention and Family Caregiver. The period of years of the journal articles was during 2006-2015.

Results: Twenty-two research-based articles met the including criteria and were included in the review. There were 14 interventional research design articles and 8 descriptive correlational research design articles recruited. There were four categories of diagnosis in this review: (I) Heart Failure (n = 3), Coronary bypass surgery (n = 1); (II) Mental Illness (n = 1), Schizophrenia and mood disorders (n = 2), Suicide (n = 1), Dementia (n = 2), Seizure (n = 1); (III) Chronic Illnesses (n = 1), Stroke (n = 3), Incapable older people and home-care services (n = 1), Diabetes (n = 1); (IV) Cancer (n = 7), Leukemia (n = 1). There were 9 countries' studies included in this review. They were Taiwan (n = 4), Canada (n = 2), Iran (n = 5), Australia (n = 1), Netherlands (n = 1), Iceland (n = 1), United States America (USA) (n = 6), German (n = 1), and

* Phone number: 816-271-4250, Email: pimingyeh@yahoo.com.

United Kingdom (UK) (n = 1). Twelve (85.71%) interventional studies had significant differences in reducing caregiver burden between pre and post test studies including Etemadifar et al. (2014), Navidian et al. (2010), Sigalet et al. (2014), Moieni et al. (2014), Sun et al. (2014), Pfeiffer et al. (2014), Northouse et al. (2013), MacNeil and Jaggers (2013), Sharif, Shaygan, and Mani (2012), Kolbrun Svavarsdottir and Olafia Sigurdardottir (2013), Pahlavanzade, Khosravi, and Moeini (2014), and Ridge et al. (2014).

Conclusion:This review highlights that interventional studies have positive effects on decreasing family caregiver's burden. The factors influencing family caregiver's burden are also described. The detail interventions of these effective randomized clinical trials (RCT) are included in this review for future studies.

Keywords: systematic review, interventions, family caregivers

INTRODUCTION

The family caregiver burden was defined as family caregiver reactions: impact on health, impact on schedule, and impact on finance (Given et al., 1992) or family perceptions including sacrifice and strain, inadequacy, embarrassment/anger, dependency, and loss of control (Zarit, Reever & Bach-Peterson, 1980). Many significant predictors of family caregiver burden have been identified among family caregivers of older people with congestive heart failure in USA (Yeh & Bull, 2009; Yeh & Bull, 2011) and among family caregivers of ill relatives with cancer, chronic illness, and stroke in Taiwan (Yeh & Chang 2011; Yeh & Chang, 2012; Yeh et al., 2009). Family caregivers play an important role to take care their loved one at hospitals or at home. There are significant differences of health status and work status between before and after being caregivers. There are many interventions that help family caregivers to relief their family caregiver burden, improve their quality of life, and psychological well-being, but few studies did a systematic review of literature of the interventions for family caregivers.

Therefore, the purpose of this study was to provide an integrative literature review of interventions for family caregivers in order to provide an evidence based information for future nursing interventions. The following review of literature was described according to the care receivers' diagnosis including interventional studies and descriptive studies.

Table 1. Characteristics of included studies
(N = 22)

Authors	*I/D	Age of care receivers (mean)	Care receivers M (%)	F (%)	Country	Care receivers' Diagnosis
Chiou et al. (2009)	D	69.6 ± 15.7 years	47.2	52.8	Taiwan	Incapable older people, stroke, and home-care services
Ducharme et al. (2014)	D				Canada	Dementia
Etemadifar et al. (2014)	I	61.09 ± 11.08 years	59.5	40.5	Iran	Heart failure

Authors	*I/D	Age of care receivers (mean)	Care receivers M (%)	F (%)	Country	Care receivers' Diagnosis
Hudson et al. (2013)	I				Australia	Advanced cancer
Joling et al. (2013)	I	Intervention group n = 96, 72.8 ± 9.1years Control group n = 96, 76.7 ± 8.3 years	68.7 66.7	31.3 33.3	Netherlands	Dementia
Kolbrun Svavarsdottir and Olafia Sigurdardottir (2013)	I	Intervention group n = 10 Average: 5.5 months (Range = 2-16 months; range for 90% children = 2-7.5 months)			Iceland	Cancer
MacNeil and Jaggers (2013)	I				USA	Serious Mental Illness
Moieni et al. (2014)	I				Iran	Coronary bypass surgery
Navidian et al. (2010)	I				Iran	Schizophrenia and mood disorders
Northouse et al. (2013)	I	*n* = 302 60.5 ± 10.9 years	38.6	61.4	USA	Cancer
Pahlavanzade, Khosravi, and Moeini (2014)	I	*Intervention group* *n* = 32, 41.5 ± 14.1 years *Control group* *n* = 32, 43.4 ± 17.07 years	56.2 65.6	48.8 34.4	Iran	Cancer (Leukemia)
Pfeiffer et al. (2014)	I	*Intervention group* *n* = 60 73.4 ± 7.5 years *Control group* *n* = 62 72.9 ± 7.5 years	69.3 69.4	31.7 30.6	German	Stroke
Ridge et al. (2014)	I	*Total N = 17* *9 female, 8 male* 13.9 ± 3 years	47.06	52.94	London, UK	Diabetes
Sharif, Shaygan, and Mani (2012)	I	*Intervention group* *n* = 33 32.5 years *Control group* *n* = 32 30 years	37 57	63 43	Iran	Schizophrenia

Table 1. (Continued)

Authors	*I/D	Age of care receivers (mean)	Care receivers M (%) F (%)		Country	Care receivers' Diagnosis
Sigalet et al. (2014)	I	Age <u>Intervention</u> <u>%</u> < 2 37.5 ≥ 2-5 54.17 ≥6-10 8.33 ≥11-17 0	<u>Control</u> <u>%</u> 24.32 51.35 8.11 16.22		Canada	Children Seizure
Sun et al. (2014)	I	*Intervention group* *n* = 37 40.5 ± 16.1 years *Control group* *n* = 37 39.7 ± 15.3 years Total Mean age: 40.1 ± 16.1	51.4 37.8 44.6	48.6 62.2 55.4	Taiwan	Suicide
Tremont, Davis, and Bishop (2006)	D	77.18 ± 9.47 years			USA	Dementia
Williams and Bakitas (2012)	D	N = 135			USA	Cancer
Yeh and Bull (2009)	D	76.47 ± 12.96 years	30	70	USA	Congestive heart failure
Yeh and Bull (2012)	D	76.47 ± 12.96 years	30	70	USA	Congestive heart failure
Yeh and Chang (2012)	D	64.92 ± 16.15 years	59.3	40.7	Taiwan	cancer, stroke, and chronic illness
Yeh, Wierenga, and Yuan (2009)	D	59.03 ± 15.59 years	62.6	37.4	Taiwan	Cancer

* I: Interventional Research Design
D: Descriptive Correlational Research Design

LITERATURE REVIEW

Category One of Diagnosis:
Heart Failure ($n = 3$) and Coronary bypass surgery ($n = 1$).

Heart Failure

Etemadifar, Bahrami, Shahriari, and Khosravi Farsani (2014) examined the effectiveness of a supportive educative group intervention on family caregiver burden of patients with heart failure. The intervention was successful in reducing caregiver burden over time both at the end of the intervention period ($p = 0.000$) and 3 months after the intervention ($p = 0.000$).

There were five sessions in this study including 1. Orientation: to increase the trustful relationship between the instructors and the family caregivers, 2. To identify the role of caregivers in health development, to understand the heart failure, and to recognize the medication of heart failure, 3. To discussion about the safety care and how to manage patient's symptom and refer the patient in an emergency situation and to indicate the importance and need to change patient's lifestyle (mobility and exercise, diet regimen, and quit smoking), 4. To promote coping strategies, problem-solving method and time management in caregiving situation, and 5. To maintain and promote caregivers' physical and mental health, as well as to increase caregivers' knowledge of supportive resources (Etemadifar et al., 2014).

This was a Randomized clinical trial (RCT) research design. There were control group and intervention group. The education team included a cardiologist physician, a psychiatric nurse, a cardiac nurse, and a clergyman. They used lecture, PowerPoint, CD, educational booklet, and phone consultation to do the education.

The Zarit Burden Interview (ZBI) was used to examine the effectiveness of this educational intervention (Etemadifar et al., 2014). The intervention group received four weekly multimedia training sessions. Every session was for 2 hours. It included education and family support and were held for four consecutive weeks (Etemadifar et al., 2014).

Yeh and Bull (2009) examined the relationships among family caregivers' spiritual well-being, coping, and mental health of family caregivers of elders with congestive heart failure. Yeh and Bull indicated that positive spiritual well-being was inversely related to negative mental health, and faith/belief systems and life satisfaction contributed to the significant correlation. Positive coping strategies were inversely related to negative mental health and the Problem Solving Coping, Alternative Perception of Events, and Dealing with Stress Symptoms contributed to the significant correlation with mental health scores (Yeh & Bull, 2009).

Yeh and Bull (2012) examined the influences of older peoples' activities of daily living dependency, family caregivers' spiritual well-being, quality of relationship, family support, coping and care continuity on the burden of family caregivers of hospitalized older people with congestive heart failure using the Resiliency Model of Family Stress, Adjustment, and Adaptation. There were 50 family caregivers and 50 older people diagnosed with congestive heart failure recruited from medical and surgical units of two Midwest medical centers. Their results indicated that there were significant positive associations between patients' activities of daily living dependence and family caregiver burden and between lack of family support and family caregiver burden. There were significant negative associations between quality of relationship and family caregiver burden, between care continuity and family caregiver burden, between coping and family caregiver burden and between spiritual well-being and burden. In hierarchical multiple regression, the model variables accounted for 66% of the variance in family caregiver burden. Patients' activities of daily living dependence, quality of relationship and lack of family support were significant predictors of family caregiver burden (Yeh & Bull, 2012).

Coronary Bypass Surgery

Moieni, Poorpooneh, and Pahlavanzadeh (2014) examined the effectiveness of family-focused nursing intervention on caregiver burden of the family members of the patients undergoing coronary bypass surgery in Isfahan Shahid Chamran Hospital during 2012. This was a clinical trial conducted on 50 family members of the patients undergoing coronary bypass surgery in Isfahan Shahid Chamran hospital. Caregivers were selected by convenient sampling and were randomly assigned to two groups of study and control. Caregivers in the study group attended a three-interventional session program during their hospitalization time, while the subjects in control group did not. Data collection tool was Novak and Guest caring burden inventory (CBI). Data were analyzed by SPSS. Caring burden before and after the intervention were $M = 30.08$ ($SD = 14.03$) and $M = 19.2$ ($SD = 10$) in the study group, respectively, and $M = 30.16$ ($SD = 12.62$) and $M = 35.44$ ($SD = 10.42$) in the control group, respectively. Changes of total scores of caring burden showed a significant difference after the intervention in the study and control groups ($p < 0.001$). Score changes of subscales of time dependence ($p < 0.001$), developmental ($p < 0.001$), physical ($p < 0.001$), and emotional caring burden ($p = 0.007$) were also significant. Results showed that family-focused nursing interventions were effective in reducing the family burden of the patients undergoing coronary bypass surgery. Nurses can administrate family-focused nursing interventions to reduce the caregiver burden (Moieni, Poorpooneh & Pahlavanzadeh, 2014).

Family intervention sessions schedule included three sessions. Session one: Educating the patients and their caregivers about the disease process as well as providing other education in order to help the caregivers to show appropriate reactions to patients' disease related problems such as pain, fatigue, and sleep and appetite disorders. Session two: Giving necessary education to help caregivers show appropriate reactions to patients' disease-related psychological and emotional problems such as anxiety, anger, depression, as well as educating the caregivers to take care of themselves. Session three: Talking to caregivers and giving them a chance to discuss about their problems and success in taking care of the patients and educating them about five steps of problem-solving skill (What is the problem? What is my plan? What might happen if? Try it out! How did I do?) and the way to use these steps to fulfill their needs concerning a caregiving role (Moieni et al., 2014).

Category Two of Diagnosis:
Mental Illness ($n = 1$), Schizophrenia and mood disorders ($n = 2$), Suicide ($n = 1$), Dementia ($n = 2$), and Seizure ($n = 1$).

Mental Illness

MacNeil and Jaggers (2013) examined the effectiveness of the Banking Positives intervention among the family caregivers of patients with serious mental illness (SMI). There were 10 family caregivers (7 female and 3 male) recruited in this study in the Alabama, USA. The results indicated that pre-test scores on the Family Burden Interview averaged 16.30, compared with 10.50 on the post-test measures ($t = 2.41$, $p = .040$). Zarit Burden Interview from a mean 51.40 at pretest to 43.50 at posttest ($t = 2.69$, $p = .025$). Therefore, there were significant improvements of relieving family caregiver burden after intervention (MacNeil & Jaggers, 2013).

The Banking Positives intervention was developed by Folkman's concept of meaning based coping to focus on the feelings of the caregivers alone, irrespective of the outcomes for the patient. The intervention is novel in that it focuses not only on positive emotions generated due to having done the right thing as a caregiver, but also on enjoyable interactions with the patient. Using a banking metaphor, the Banking Positives intervention uses elements of cognitive therapy to help family caregivers to generate positive emotions in coping situations. Specifically, it helps caregivers to become aware of their cognitive and emotional perceptions of their caregiving relationship (capital), challenging negative thoughts, focusing on the positive thoughts and emotions associated with their caregiving (banking them), accessing these positive thoughts and feelings when confronted by caregiving challenges (using capital), and applying this process to other issues that confront them as family caregivers, such as future planning for their relative.

Schizophrenia and Mood Disorders

Navidian, Pahlavanzadeh, and Yazdani (2010) evaluated the effectiveness of a group psycho-educational program on family caregivers of inpatients with mental disorders in Isfahan. This was a single blind randomized clinical trial. One hundred family caregivers of psychiatric inpatients were recruited in this study for three months. Family caregiver burden was assessed by Zarit Burden Interview. The mean score of burden in family care givers of patients with schizophrenia and mood disorders significantly decreased ($p = 0.001$) in comparison with the control group. The group intervention program for reducing family caregivers burden was effective (Navidian, Pahlavanzadeh & Yazdani, 2010). The content of this article was not in English. It was in Iran language.

Sharif, Shaygan, and Mani (2012) examined the effectiveness of family psycho-education in reducing patients' symptoms and on family caregiver burden. Sixty five Iranian outpatients with a diagnosis of schizophrenia disorder and their caregivers were randomly allocated to the experimental ($n = 33$) or control groups ($n = 32$). Patients in the experimental group received antipsychotic drug treatment and a psycho-educational program was arranged for their caregivers. The psycho-educational program consisted of ten 90-min sessions held during five weeks (two sessions in each week). Each caregiver attended 10 sessions (in five weeks). At baseline, immediately after intervention, and one month later, validated tools were used to assess patients' clinical status and caregiver burden. Compared with the control group, the experimental group showed significantly reduced symptom severity and caregiver burden both immediately after intervention and one month later. These results suggest that even need based short-term psycho-educational intervention for family members of Iranian patients with schizophrenic disorder may improve the outcomes of patients and their families (Sharif, Shaygan & Mani, 2012).

Suicide

Sun, Chiang, Lin, and Chen (2014) examined the short-term effects of a suicide care educational intervention on the family's ability to care, family's caring stress levels and family's attitudes towards attempted suicide. This was an experimental design, using two groups and a pre- and post-intervention survey was used. A randomized controlled study was conducted with 74 family caregivers of people who are suicidal (37 using suicide education and 37 in the control group). The experimental group was provided with a two-hour suicide care education intervention, and the control group received normal suicide care support. Participants were recruited at a Suicide Prevention Centre and two acute psychiatric hospitals. Three questionnaires were collected: (1) the Suicidal Caring Ability Scale (2) the Caring Stress Scale and (3) the Suicide Attitudes Scale. The results demonstrated that there were statistically significant differences in the Suicidal Caring Ability Scale and the Suicide Attitudes Scale but no statistically significant differences in the Caring Stress Scale. That is, the suicide education program can promote the ability to care for people who are suicidal and can generate a positive attitude towards people who are suicidal from their caregivers. Therefore, clinical practice Nurses could use the two-hour personal suicidal education program to increase one's ability to care for their relatives who had attempted suicide and promote one's positive attitudes towards attempted suicide (Sun, Chiang, Lin & Chen, 2014).

Suicide education program included to ensure that all sites received the same program, a standard suicide education protocol was developed. First, the research team designed an educational handbook for families dealing with suicide. The contents of the handbook followed the methods of Sun and Long (2008), who developed a theory for caring for suicidal people for caregivers. A characteristic of the suicide education handbook was its easy-to-understand explanations that include narratives and statements about real experiences of families of people who are suicidal. The 40-page suicide education handbook was written by the researchers and was entitled 'Mind Helper — How to Assist Family Members Dealing with Suicide'. It is four chapters long and contains one appendix. The content of the chapters and appendix are as follows: The objectives of the first chapter, understanding suicide, were to help family members become aware of the emotional pain that suicidal people experience and to inform them of some of the known reasons why people experience this pain and anguish. It includes definitions of suicide, the epidemiology of suicide, the reasons for suicide and philosophical debates concerning the meaning and value of life. The purpose of the second chapter, the environment of caring for people who are suicidal, was to decrease the disgrace related to suicide and suicidal behaviors in their society and to help family members seek early treatment for their suicidal relatives. It includes sections on teaching family members healthy attitudes towards suicide and on caregiver stress in their culture. The objectives of the third chapter, the effects of family care, were to help family members improve the care that they were providing. It included information on support systems, families' coping strategies, difficulties with care and problems with a family's ability to provide care. The fourth chapter, skills in caring for people at risk for suicide, aims to increase family caregivers' ability to care for their suicidal relatives, promote their physical recovery and facilitate their mental healing. It includes information on assessing suicide risk, creating a safe environment, teaching family members to use open and effective communication to relieve distress in suicidal people, helping suicidal people comply with medication regimes and teaching positive thinking strategies to re-awaken hope in people who are suicidal. The appendix was added at the end of the handbook to provide suicide prevention resources, for example, the Internet addresses, mailing addresses, and telephone numbers of mental health consultant institutions, hospitals and societal resources (Sun et al., 2014).

Suicide care educational intervention with the guidance of the suicide education handbook (Sun et al., 2014). The intervention included the following:

1. Two hours of formal personal instruction using the suicide education handbook: A researcher who is a psychiatric nursing teachers in the university and has psychiatric nursing experiences for over 15 years and a RA provided the handbook and spent two hours explaining the contents of the handbook and discussing patients' experiences with suicide care either in the hospital or at the family's home.
2. Two individual follow-up consultations by telephone with a family researcher or RA: The family caregivers of people who are suicidal would clarify their problems concerning suicide care during two follow-up consultations, with the first follow-up taking place within one week following the two hours of formal personal instruction. The second follow-up took place within two months of the first follow-up.
3. Free telephone consultations with a family researcher or RA: Family caregivers suffer many difficulties when they care for suicidal relatives. Therefore, the researcher who teaches counseling theory and practice in the university and has done suicide research for 15 years or RAs left their telephone numbers with participating family caregivers to encourage continued consultation about their difficulties (Sun et al., 2014).

Dementia

Joling et al. (2013) examined the effectiveness of family meetings intervention to prevent depression and anxiety in family caregivers of patients with dementia. The research design was a randomized trial. Dementia imposes a heavy burden on health and social care systems as well as on family caregivers who provide a substantial portion of the care. Interventions that effectively support caregivers may prevent or delay patient institutionalization and hence be cost-effective. However, evidence about the cost-effectiveness of such interventions is scarce. Joling et al. evaluated the cost-effectiveness of a family meetings intervention for family caregivers of dementia patients in comparison with usual care over a period of 12 months. The economic evaluation was conducted from a societal perspective alongside a randomized trial of 192 primary caregivers with community-dwelling dementia patients. Outcome measures included the Quality Adjusted Life-Years (QALY) of caregivers and patients and the incidence of depression and anxiety disorders in caregivers. Missing cost and effect data were imputed using multiple imputations. Bootstrapping was used to estimate uncertainty around the cost-differences and the incremental cost-effectiveness ratio (ICER). The bootstrapped cost-effect pairs were plotted on a cost-effectiveness plane and used to estimate cost-effectiveness curves. No significant differences in costs and effects between the groups were found. At 12 months, total costs per patient and primary caregiver dyad were substantial: 77,832 for the intervention group and 75,201 for the usual care group (adjusted mean difference per dyad 4,149, 95% CI -13,371 to 21,956, ICER 157,534). The main cost driver was informal care (66% of total costs), followed by patients' day treatment and costs of hospital and long-term care facility admissions (23%). Based on the cost-effectiveness acceptability curves, the maximum probability that the intervention was considered cost-effective in comparison with usual care reached 0.4 for the outcome QALY per patient-caregiver dyad and 0.6 for the caregivers' incidence of depression and/or anxiety disorders regardless of the willingness to pay. Therefore, the annual costs of caring for a person with dementia were substantial with informal care being by far the largest contributor to the total societal costs. Based on this study, family meetings cannot be considered a cost-effective intervention strategy in comparison with usual care.

Tremont, Davis, and Bishop (2006) examined the interrelationships between family functioning, caregiver burden, and patient characteristics. Seventy-two family caregivers who lived with care receivers with mild ($n = 47$) or moderate dementia ($n = 25$) were recruited in this study. Their results indicated that higher levels of caregiver burden were significantly associated with increased caregiver depression and anxiety, greater frequency of memory and behavior problems in the dementia patient, worse activities of daily living, and poorer family functioning. Caregivers with high levels of burden reported greater family dysfunction in communication and roles, regardless of their relationship to the patient (i.e., spouse or child) (Tremont, Davis & Bishop, 2006).

Ducharme et al. (2014) used a mixed research design to examine the unmet support needs of early-onset dementia family caregivers. Participants were 32 family caregivers in their 50s recruited through memory clinics and Alzheimer Societies in Quebec (Canada). The Family Caregivers Support Agreement (FCSA) tool was used to collect data combined with open-ended questions. Their results indicated that 70% of the caregivers reported unmet support needs that were primarily of a psycho-educational nature. Caregivers wished primarily: (1) to receive more information on available help and financial resources; (2) to have their relatives feel valued as persons and to offer them stimulating activities adjusted to their residual abilities; (3) to reduce stress stemming from their caregiver role assumed at an early age and to have the chance to enjoy more time for themselves; and (4) to receive help at the right time and for the help to be tailored to their situation of caregiver of a young person.

Seizure

Sigalet et al. (2014) examined the effectiveness of simulation-based seizure management teaching on improving caregiver competence and reported confidence with managing seizures. The authors hypothesized that simulation-based education would lead to a higher level of demonstrated competence and reported confidence in family members and caregivers. A two-group pre- and post-test experimental research design involving a total of 61 caregivers was used. The intervention was a simulation-based seizure curriculum delivered as a supplement to traditional seizure discharge teaching. Caregiver performance was analyzed using a seizure management checklist. Caregivers' perception of self-efficacy was evaluated by a self-efficacy questionnaire. Caregivers in the experimental group achieved significantly higher postintervention performance scores than caregivers in the control group in both premedication and postmedication seizure management ($p < 0.01$). Additionally, they achieved significantly higher scores on the self-efficacy questionnaire including items reflecting confidence managing the seizure at home ($p < 0.05$) (Sigalet et al., 2014).

Category Three of Diagnosis:

Chronic Illnesses ($n = 1$), Stroke ($n = 3$), Incapable older people and home-care services ($n = 1$), and Diabetes ($n = 1$).

Chronic Illnesses

Yeh and Chang (2012) examined the relationships among family caregivers' reactions and their related factors among Taiwanese with hospitalized relatives. In Taiwan, most hospitalized patients have relatives or foreign laborers with them 24 hours a day. A convenience sample of 200 primary caregivers of hospitalized patients diagnosed with cancer, stroke, and chronic illness was recruited. Their results indicated that participants with a moderate level of family support experienced a moderate impact on health and finances, but a high impact on schedule. Family caregivers' health status and work time were significantly different between, before and after serving as a family caregiver. The multiple regression model variables accounted for 40.1% of the total family caregivers' reaction variance. Three factors were found to predict significantly greater impact on a family caregiver: (1) lower scores of caregiving knowledge, (2) increasing patient's activities of daily living dependency and (3) lack of family support.

Stroke

Pfeiffer et al. (2014) examined the effectiveness the telephone-based problem-solving intervention (PSI) for family caregivers of stroke survivors after the early poststroke period. This was a randomized controlled trial. The including criteria of family caregivers were who provided care for at least 6 months and who experienced significant strain in their role. One hundred twenty-two family caregivers (age = 66.2 years, 77.9% female) were randomly allocated to a PSI or control group.

The PSI was composed of 2 home visits and 18 telephone calls delivered over a 3-month intensive intervention and a 9-month maintenance period. PSI and control groups received monthly information letters in addition to usual care. Primary caregiver outcomes were depressive symptoms (measure: Center for Epidemiologic Studies–Depression Scale) and sense of competence (measure:

Sense of Competence Questionnaire). Their results indicated that caregivers of the PSI group showed significantly lower levels of depressive symptoms after 3 months ($p < .01$, $d = -.48$) and after 12 months ($p < .05$, $d = -.37$), but no better sense of competence compared with the control group. Latent growth curve analyses revealed positive significant ($p < .05$) linear and quadratic effects of PSI on both primary outcomes (Pfeiffer et al., 2014).

Incapable Older People and Home-Care Services

Chiou, Chang, Chen, and Wang (2009) investigated the association between perceived and received social support and caregiver burden among 301 family caregivers in Taiwan. The caregivers were caring for ill or incapable family members, who were clients of home-care services in Taiwan. Caregiver burden was likely to be higher when the caregivers had lower levels of family function and social support. Perceived social support was better at predicting caregiver burden than received social support. The results of this study indicated that family function had an important influence on caregiver burden. According to the results, family based interventions are needed to determine approaches for effectively reducing caregiver burden (Chiou, Chang, Chen & Wang, 2009).

Diabetes

Ridge et al. (2014) examined the effectiveness of Diabetes-Oriented Learning Family Intervention (DOLFIN) for caregivers of young persons with Type 1 diabetes. Participants were caregivers of young persons aged 10-18 years with a diagnosis of Type 1 diabetes of more than 12 months' duration in two inner-city South London hospitals. Caregivers were invited to attend six sessions of a group workshop where they received emotional support, diabetes education and were taught motivational interviewing techniques to support their child. Their results indicated that out of 106 eligible participants, caregivers of 31 young people with Type 1 diabetes were recruited, 17 of whom 'completed' the intervention (attending four or more sessions). Participants discussed a variety of themes in session, including the increasing difficulty of diabetes management as children grow older, parenting techniques for managing diabetes in the home and the emotional challenges of having a child with a chronic illness. Engaging parents in a caregiver intervention for Type 1 diabetes was a challenge, but parents who participated appeared to value the program. Future interventions for caregiver need to take account of caregivers' wishes and expectations in order to maximize user uptake (Ridge et al., 2014). The Diabetes-Oriented Learning Family Intervention (DOLFIN): 1. involve parents in diabetes care whilst respecting clinic recommendations for adolescent independence; 2. empower carers as collaborators in diabetes management; 3. increase positive interactions between parent and child (Ridge et al., 2014).

Ridge et al. described that DOLFIN used animal metaphors to describe some of the natural, instinctive parenting styles that can emerge when caring for a loved one with an illness. These metaphors illustrate adaptive and maladaptive relationship patterns; including a jellyfish with intense and sometimes painful emotional reactions, an ostrich who might seek comfort by denying problems and putting their head in the sand, a terrier who uses an insistent approach to get their point across, a kangaroo who takes on all roles and can be overly protective by keeping someone in their pouch, and an overly directive rhinoceros who demands change. A dolphin was used to describe an 'optimal' caring style, epitomizing a carer who sometimes swims in front of a young person leading the way, other times encouragingly alongside and sometimes quietly behind. Animal metaphors enabled light-hearted and non-judgemental group discussion of the topic of expressed emotions and parenting styles in diabetes. Motivational interviewing was used as a framework to practice 'dolphin-like behaviour' and techniques for sidestepping expressed emotions and increasing positive interactions were explored (Ridge et al., 2014).

Category Four of Diagnosis
Cancer ($n = 7$) and Leukemia ($n = 1$).

Cancer

Northouse et al. (2013) examined (i) whether patient-caregiver dyads (i.e., pairs) randomly assigned to a brief or extensive dyadic intervention (the FOCUS Program) had better outcomes, quality of life (QOL), than dyads randomly assigned to usual care and (ii) whether patients' risk for distress and other factors moderated the effect of the brief or extensive program on outcomes. Advanced cancer patients and their caregivers ($N = 484$ dyads) were stratified by patients' baseline risk for distress (high versus low), cancer type (lung, colorectal, breast, or prostate), and research site and then randomly assigned to a brief (three-session) or extensive (six-session) intervention or control. The interventions offered dyads information and support. Intermediary outcomes were appraisals (i.e., appraisal of illness/caregiving, uncertainty, and hopelessness) and resources (i.e., coping, interpersonal relationships, and self-efficacy). The primary outcome was QOL. Data were collected prior to intervention and post-intervention (3 and 6 months from baseline). The final sample was 302 dyads. Repeated measures MANCOVA was used to evaluate outcomes. The results indicated that there was a significant improvement in dyads' coping ($p < 0.05$), self-efficacy ($p < 0.05$), and social QOL ($p < 0.01$) and in caregivers' emotional QOL ($p < 0.05$). Effects varied by intervention dose. Most effects were found at 3 months only. Risk for distress accounted for very few moderation effects. Therefore, both brief and extensive programs had positive outcomes for patient-caregiver dyads, but few sustained effects (Northouse et al., 2013).

Kolbrun Svavarsdottir and Olafia Sigurdardottir (2013) examined the effectiveness of a two-to-three session family therapeutic conversation intervention (FAM-TCI) for primary and partner caregivers of children and adolescents in active cancer treatment on perceived family support and on expressive family functioning. This was a quasi-experimental research design. There was one group pre and post-test. The participants were recruited from inpatient cancer unit and a day treatment cancer unit at the Children's Hospital in Reykjavik, Iceland. There were 19 parent caregivers (10 primary, 9 partner) of children in active cancer medical treatment. The caregivers completed baseline measure questionnaires and were offered the first sessions of the FAM-TCI. About four to eight weeks later, the second session was administered and then the caregivers were offered a third session, if needed, one week later. When the caregivers had finished all sessions, they answered the same set of questionnaires about one week later. The main research variables were the FAM-TCI for primary and partner caregivers, family support, and expressive family functioning. Their results indicated that primary caregivers perceived significantly higher family support after the intervention compared to before. Those caregivers also reported significantly higher expressive family functioning and significantly higher emotional communication after the intervention. Partner caregivers, however, reported significantly lower verbal communication after the FAM-TCI compared to before (Kolbrun Svavarsdottir & Olafia Sigurdardottir, 2013).

Hudson et al. (2013) examined the effectiveness of psycho-educational intervention on caregivers for the role of supporting a patient with advanced cancer receiving home-based palliative care. Their hypothesis was that primary family caregivers who participated in the intervention would report decreased psychological distress (primary outcome), fewer unmet needs and increased levels of perceived preparedness, competence and positive emotions. A three-arm randomized controlled trial was conducted comparing two versions of the intervention (one face-to-face visit versus two visits) plus standard care to a control group (standard care) across four sites in Australia. Their results indicated that a total of 298 participants were recruited; 148 were in the control condition, 57 in intervention 1 (one visit) and 93 in intervention 2 (two visits). Relative to participants in the control group; the psychological well-being of participants in the intervention condition was improved by a small amount but non-significantly. No significant reduction in unmet needs or improvements in positive aspects of caregiving amongst the intervention group were identified. However, the intervention demonstrated significant improvements in participants' levels of preparedness and competence for intervention 2 (Hudson et al., 2013).

Hudson et al. (2013) indicated that the psycho-educational focus included tailored information and resources given to family caregivers to promote psychological well-being by preparing them for their role. Each caregiver was allocated a Family Caregiver Support Nurse (FCSN) who assisted the local palliative care service to assess caregiver needs, establish a care plan and provide additional caregiver support. The FCSNs (one per recruitment site) received training from relevant members of the research team and an intervention manual was developed to foster consistency in delivery. The primary written resource was a family caregiver guidebook, developed and tested in our pilot work. The intervention was delivered over 4 weeks and comprised the following: Step 1 involved preparing caregivers for the intervention. The FCSN (i) phoned family caregivers within 3 days of randomization to advise them of the FCSN role; (ii) sent them the family caregiver guidebook; (iii) provided written information about the FCSN/the intervention; and (iv) arranged a home visit within 1 week. Step 2 involved assessing caregiver needs and preparing a care plan. Home visit was carried out by the FCSN who (i) assessed unmet needs; (ii) developed a care plan in conjunction with the caregiver (and the patient, where pertinent) and the local palliative care team; and (iii) prepared the caregivers for their role by explaining educational resources. Step 3 involved re-assessing needs and evaluating the care plan: The FCSN reviewed caregivers' status and evaluated the care plan by phone. Caregivers were reminded about relevant resources and strategies to promote psychological well-being, including trying to identify positive aspects of caring. Step 4 involved assisting the family caregiver to prepare for their relative's death and to prepare for bereavement. Home visit by the FCSN was carried out to focus on preparing caregiver for aspects typically associated with imminent death. Caregivers were also advised of common reactions during bereavement and of available bereavement resources. The FCSN concluded the structured component of the intervention with a summary (including written format) of key strategies and resources (Hudson et al., 2013).

Yeh, Wierenga, and Yuan (2009) examined the influences of psychological well-being, quality of caregiver-patient relationship, and family support on the health of family caregivers for cancer patients in a Taiwanese hospital. Ninety one family caregivers of hospitalized cancer patients completed the Caregiver Reaction Assessment and Psychological Well-Being Scale. Their results indicated that the psychological well-being and the quality of the caregiver-patient relationship of family caregivers were found to be significantly positively correlated with caregivers' health. The lack of family support was found to be significantly negatively correlated with caregivers' health. Psychological well-being, quality of caregiver-patient relationship, and family support accounted for 59% of the variance in caregivers' health (Yeh, Wierenga & Yuan, 2009).

Williams and Bakitas (2012) explored the lived experience of being a caregiver for an adult with lung or colon cancer in order to develop future intervention studies. This was a phenomenological research design and the open-ended interviews were conducted at a chemotherapy clinic, New Haven, CT with 135 caregivers of patients with lung or colon cancer. Interviews were audio-recorded and transcribed. Thematic analysis was conducted with transcripts coded, reviewed, and recoded multiple times. The final 69 codes were reduced to 13 code clusters (thematic categories) distributed among 4 themes. Their results indicated that four inter-related themes emerged: 1) becoming a caregiver; 2) new and altered relationships; 3) personal responses to caregiving and 4) antecedents and social context. Caregivers describe hearing the cancer diagnosis as 'life-changing'. The cancer creates the context for the caregiver's relationships (with the patient, self, others, and the healthcare system), and cognitive, behavioral, affective, and spiritual responses.

The caregiver's antecedent experiences and social support network form the foundation for their perceptions of the diagnosis, relationships, and personal responses (Williams & Bakitas, 2012).

Leukemia

Pahlavanzade, Khosravi, and Moeini (2014) examined the effectiveness of a family need-based program on the burden of care in caregivers of leukemia patients. In this clinical research, 70 caregivers of leukemia patients who referred to Sayed Al-Shohada Medical Center in Isfahan, Iran were chosen and divided, through convenient sampling method and using table of random numbers, into two groups, experimental and control. Caregivers of the experimental group attended five training sessions.

The data collection tool of this study was the Zarit Burden Scale. It was completed by members of both groups before, immediately after, and 1 month after the intervention.

The data obtained were analyzed with SPSS software. Their results indicated that during the study period, burden slowly decreased in the experimental group and increased in the control group. Mean burden of care score before, immediately after, and 1 month after the intervention was 63.6, 30.4, and 23.03, respectively, in the experimental group and 62.5, 67.3, and 68.8, respectively, in the control group. In addition, the mean burden score in the experimental group significantly decreased in comparison with the control group ($P < 0.001$).

Therefore, this family need-based program can decrease burden in caregivers of leukemia patients and may potentially improve the quality of life of both patients and caregivers (Pahlavanzade, Khosravi & Moeini, 2014).

Pahlavanzade, Khosravi, and Moeini's Training program content is summarized as follows:

First session: Introducing the caregivers to the researcher and setting plans and goals, and question and answer.

Second session: Providing information on leukemia, the complications after medication therapy, and importance of follow-up and care of patients.

Third session: Providing information about self-care, and strengthening the social dimension and social interactions of the caregivers.

Fourth session: Providing information on problem-solving skills and techniques to reduce stress and anxiety in caregivers.

Fifth session: Strengthening their spiritual dimension. In the final session, a CD containing relaxation, and stress and anger management techniques, and educational booklets on the content of each session in summary were prepared and provided for the study subjects.

Furthermore, for spiritual intervention, a religious expert helped. In addition, for 1 month after the intervention, the experimental group members were given advice based on their needs via telephone, and if needed, they were referred to the assistance unit or psychiatrist specialists. The caregivers of the control group did not participate in this program. However, at the end of the intervention, the CDs and booklets were left at their disposal (Pahlavanzade, Khosravi & Moeini, 2014).

METHODS

Design

This was an integrative review research design.

Data Collection and Analysis

The peer-reviewed journal articles were searched from the following databases: Academic Search Complete, Academic Search Premier, CINAHL, MEDLINE, and PsycINFO. The key words were Intervention and Family Caregiver.

The period of years of the journal articles was during 2006-2015. The inclusion criteria for study selection were their abstract published in English and appeared in refereed journals. The literature was reviewed and analyzed according to the care receivers' diagnosis, countries, interventional studies, and descriptive correlational studies. Their effectiveness of interventions and interventional strategies were analyzed. The important factors influencing family caregiver burden were also described in this review article.

RESULTS

Twenty-two research-based articles met the including criteria and were included in the review. There were 14 interventional research design articles and 8 descriptive correlational research design articles were recruited. There were four categories of diagnosis in this review: (I) Heart Failure ($n = 3$), Coronary bypass surgery ($n = 1$); (II) Mental Illness ($n = 1$), Schizophrenia and mood disorders ($n = 2$), Suicide ($n = 1$), Dementia ($n = 2$), Seizure ($n = 1$); (III) Chronic Illnesses ($n = 1$), Stroke ($n = 3$), Incapable older people and home-care services ($n = 1$), Diabetes ($n = 1$); (IV) Cancer ($n = 7$), Leukemia ($n = 1$).

There were 9 countries' studies included in this review. They were Taiwan ($n = 4$), Canada ($n = 2$), Iran ($n = 5$), Australia ($n = 1$), Netherlands ($n = 1$), Iceland ($n = 1$), United States America (USA) ($n = 6$), German ($n = 1$), and United Kingdom (UK) ($n = 1$). Twelve

(85.71%) interventional studies had significant differences in reducing caregiver burden between pre and post test studies including Etemadifar et al. (2014), Navidian et al. (2010), Sigalet et al. (2014), Moieni et al. (2014), Sun et al. (2014), Pfeiffer et al. (2014), Northouse et al. (2013), MacNeil and Jaggers (2013), Sharif, Shaygan, and Mani (2012), Kolbrun Svavarsdottir and Olafia Sigurdardottir (2013), Pahlavanzade, Khosravi, and Moeini (2014), and Ridge et al. (2014).

Highlight these successful interventional researches to decrease family caregiver burden were described as follows. Etemadifar et al. (2014) examined the effectiveness of *a supportive educative group intervention* on family caregiver burden of patients with heart failure. The intervention was successful in reducing caregiver burden over time both at the end of the intervention period ($p = 0.000$) and 3 months after the intervention ($p = 0.000$).

There were five sessions in this study. Etemadifar et al. provided very detailed interventional strategies and kept following up their participants. *Zarit Burden Interview* was used to measure the family caregiver's burden. Navidian et al. (2010) evaluated the effectiveness of *a group psycho-educational program* on family caregivers of inpatients with mental disorders in Isfahan. Family caregiver burden was assessed by *Zarit Burden Interview*. The mean score of burden in family care givers of patients with schizophrenia and mood disorders significantly decreased ($p = 0.001$) in comparison with the control group.

Sigalet et al. (2014) examined the effectiveness of simulation-based seizure management teaching on improving caregiver competence and reported confidence with managing seizures. The intervention was a *simulation-based seizure curriculum* delivered as a supplement to traditional seizure discharge teaching. Caregivers in the experimental group achieved significantly higher post-intervention performance scores than caregivers in the control group in both pre-medication and post-medication seizure management ($p < 0.01$). Additionally, they achieved significantly higher scores on the self-efficacy questionnaire including items reflecting confidence managing the seizure at home ($p < 0.05$) (Sigalet et al., 2014).

Moieni et al. (2014) examined the effectiveness of *family-focused nursing intervention on caregiver burden* of the family members of the patients undergoing coronary bypass surgery in Isfahan Shahid Chamran Hospital during 2012. This was a clinical trial conducted on 50 family members of the patients undergoing coronary bypass surgery in Isfahan Shahid Chamran hospital. Caregivers were selected by convenient sampling and were randomly assigned to two groups of study and control. Caregivers in the study group attended a three-interventional session program during their hospitalization time, while the subjects in control group did not. Data collection tool was *Novak and Guest caring burden inventory (CBI)*. Changes of total scores of caring burden showed a significant difference after the intervention in the study and control groups ($p < 0.001$). Score changes of subscales of time dependence ($p < 0.001$), developmental ($p < 0.001$), physical ($p < 0.001$), and emotional caring burden ($p = 0.007$) were also significant. Results showed that family-focused nursing interventions were effective in reducing the family burden of the patients undergoing coronary bypass surgery (Moieni, Poorpooneh & Pahlavanzadeh, 2014).

Table 2. Summary of the studies of interventions for family caregivers (n = 14)

Authors	Design	Family Caregivers	Intervention	Instrument	Findings
Etemadifar et al. (2014)	Randomized clinical trial (RCT)	*Intervention group* n = 42, 76.2% female 40.78 ± 9.30 years *Control group* n = 45, 84.4% female 41.44 ± 9.21 years	Supportive educative group; four weekly multimedia training sessions of 2 h that included education and family support	Zarit Burden Interview (ZBI)	The intervention was successful in reducing caregiver burden over time both at the end of the intervention period (p = 0.000) and 3 months after the intervention (p = 0.000).
Navidian et al. (2010)	Randomized clinical trial (RCT)	100 family caregivers of psychiatric inpatients	A group psycho-educational program	Zarit Burden Interview (ZBI)	The mean score of burden in family care givers of patients with schizophrenia and mood disorders significantly decreased (p = 0.001) in comparison with the control group.
Sigalet et al. (2014)	Randomized clinical trial (RCT)	*Intervention group* n = 24, 50% male *Control group* n = 37, 62.16% male	A simulation-based seizure management teaching program	The new KidSIM-ASPIRE Emergent Seizure Management Checklist, The KidSIM-ASPIRE Parent Seizure Self-efficacy Questionnaire	Caregivers in the experimental group achieved significantly higher post-intervention performance scores and the scores of self-efficacy questionnaire than caregivers in the control group.
Moieni et al. (2014)	Randomized clinical trial (RCT)	*Intervention group* n = 25, 96% female 40.4 ± 10 years *Control group* n = 25, 88% female 37.8 ± 8.9 years	Family-focused nursing intervention on caregiver burden	Novak and Guest caregiver burden inventory	Results showed that family-focused nursing interventions were effective in reducing the family burden of the patients undergoing coronary bypass surgery.

Authors	Design	Family Caregivers	Intervention	Instrument	Findings
					Caring burden before and after the intervention were $M = 30.08$ ($SD = 14.03$) and $M = 19.2$ ($SD = 10$).
Sun et al. (2014)	Randomized clinical trial (RCT)	*Intervention group* $n = 37$, 73% female 49.8 ± 13.1 years *Control group* $n = 37$, 48.6% female 41.0 ± 12.4 years	A suicide care educational intervention on the family's ability, stress, and attitudes	The Suicidal Caring Ability Scale, the Caring Stress Scale, and the Suicidal Attitudes Scale	The results demonstrated that there were statistically significant differences in the Suicidal Caring Ability Scale and the Suicide Attitudes Scale but no statistically significant differences in the Caring Stress Scale.
Pfeiffer et al. (2014)	Randomized clinical trial (RCT)	*Intervention group* $n = 60$, 76.7% female 66.7 ± 9.9 years *Control group* $n = 62$, 79% female 65.6 ± 10.1 years	Telephone-based problem-solving intervention	Center for Epidemiologic Studies–Depression Scale, Sense of Competence Questionnaire	PSI group showed significantly lower levels of depressive symptoms after 3 months and after 12 months, but no better sense of competence compared with the control group.
Northouse et al. (2013)	Randomized clinical trial (RCT)	*Total:* $n = 302$, 55.8% female 56.7 ± 12.6 years *Intervention group* $n = 99$ (extensive session) $n = 99$ (brief session) *Control group* $n = 104$	FOCUS Program, a brief (three-session) or extensive (six-session) intervention	Omega Clinical Screening Interview (Risk for distress), Appraisal of Illness Scale (patients) and Appraisal of Caregiving Scale (caregivers), a brief version of the Mishel Uncertainty in Illness Scale (Uncertainty),	The results indicated that there was a significant improvement in dyads' coping ($p < 0.05$), self-efficacy ($p < 0.05$), and social QOL ($p < 0.01$) and in caregivers' emotional QOL ($p < 0.05$).

Table 2. (Continued)

Authors	Design	Family Caregivers	Intervention	Instrument	Findings
				Beck Hopelessness Scale (Hopelessness), Brief Cope (Coping Strategies), Healthy behaviors scale, Social Support Questionnaire, Lewis Mutuality and Sensitivity Scale, Lewis Cancer Self-efficacy Scale, the general Functional Assessment of Cancer Therapy (Quality of life).	
MacNeil and Jaggers (2013)	A convenience sampling strategy, pre and post tests	n = 10, 70% female 66 years (Range: 58-80 years)	The Banking Positives intervention	The assistance in daily living module of the Family Burden Interview Schedule–Short Form, The Centers for Epidemiologic Studies Depression Scale, the Zarit Burden Interview, The Philadelphia Geriatric Center Positive Affect Scale,	Pre-test scores on the Family Burden Interview averaged 16.30, compared with 10.50 on the post-test measures (t = 2.41, p = .040). Zarit Burden Interview from a mean 51.40 at pretest to 43.50 at posttest (t = 2.69, p = .025).

Authors	Design	Family Caregivers	Intervention	Instrument	Findings
				Positive Aspects of Caregiving instrument, Quality of Life Inventory, Modified Caregiver Strain Index	
Joling et al. (2013)	Randomized clinical trial (RCT)	*Intervention group* $n = 96$, 69.8% female 67.8 ± 9.8 years *Control group* $n = 96$, 70.8% female 71.2 ± 10.7 years	Family meetings intervention	HADS-A: Hospital Anxiety and Depression Scales-Anxiety subscale; CES-D: Centre for Epidemiologic Studies Depression Scale; (I) ADL: (Instrumental) activities of daily living; MMSE: Mini Mental State Examination.	No significant differences in costs and effects between the groups
Sharif, Shaygan, and Mani (2012)	Randomized clinical trial (RCT)	*Intervention group* $n = 33$ 50.5 years *Control group* $n = 32$ 52.5 years The majority of caregivers in both groups were mothers of patients	Family psycho-education intervention	Iranian version of the Brief Psychiatric Rating Scale (BPRS), Family Burden questionnaire	Compared with the control group, the experimental group showed significantly reduced symptom severity and caregiver burden both immediately after intervention and one month later.

Table 2. (Continued)

Authors	Design	Family Caregivers	Intervention	Instrument	Findings
Kolbrun Svavarsdottir and Olafia Sigurdardottir (2013)	Quasi-experimental research design	*Intervention group* n = 10, 90% Female 31-40 years (60%) 41-50 years (30%) 51-60 years (10%)	Therapeutic Conversation Intervention	Iceland Family Perceived Support Questionnaire (ICE-FPSQ) and the Iceland Expressive Family Functioning Questionnaire (ICE-EFFQ).	Their results indicated that primary caregivers perceived significantly higher family support after the intervention compared to before. Those caregivers also reported significantly higher expressive family functioning and significantly higher emotional communication after the intervention.
Pahlavanzade, Khosravi, and Moeini (2014)	Randomized clinical trial (RCT)	*Intervention group* n = 32, 71.9% female 39.1 ± 9.6 years *Control group* n = 32, 51.4% female 40.3 ± 12.1 years	Family need-based program on burden of caregivers of leukemia patients	Zarit Burden Scale	Mean burden of care score before, immediately after, and 1 month after the intervention was 63.6, 30.4, and 23.03, respectively, in the experimental group and 62.5, 67.3, and 68.8, respectively, in the control group. The mean burden score in the experimental group significantly decreased in comparison with the control group ($P < 0.001$).

Authors	Design	Family Caregivers	Intervention	Instrument	Findings
Hudson et al. (2013)	Randomized clinical trial (RCT)	*Total N = 298* 59 ± 13.9 years (Range 22-88 years) Male: 61.7 Female: 57.9 *Intervention group 1* *n* = 57, 70% female *Intervention group 2* *n* = 93, 75% female *Control group* *n* = 148, 70% female	Psycho-educational intervention to decrease family caregivers' psychological distress	General Health Questionnaire, Caregiver Competence Scale, Preparedness for Caregiving Scale, Family Inventory of Need—Part/Scale, Rewards for Caregiving Scale	No significant improvement on family caregiver's psychological well-being and no significant reduction in unmet needs or improvements in positive aspects of caregiving amongst the intervention group
Ridge et al. (2014)	Quasi-experimental research design, pilot study	*Total N = 17* *15 female, 2 male* 45.4 ± 8.8 years	Diabetes-Oriented Learning Family Intervention (DOLFIN)	*Child measures:* Diabetes Family Conflict Scale, Diabetes Family Responsibility Questionnaire. *Carer measures:* Patient Health Questionnaire, Generalized Anxiety Disorder, Diabetes Family Conflict Scale, Diabetes Family Responsibility Questionnaire.	Four Themes: 1. Adjusting to change, 2. Knowledge: 'What should I do?' 3. Emotional ventilation: 'You never get over it' 4. Self recognition: 'I think I'm a bit of a kangaroo The authors did not showed the statistic differences between pre-and post tests. They showed the mean differences.

Sun et al. (2014) examined the short-term effects of a *suicide care educational intervention* on the family's ability to care, family's caring stress levels and family's attitudes towards attempted suicide.

The experimental group was provided with a two-hour suicide care education intervention, and the control group received normal suicide care support. Three questionnaires were collected: (1) the Suicidal Caring Ability Scale (2) the Caring Stress Scale and (3) the Suicide Attitudes Scale. The results demonstrated that there were statistically significant differences in the Suicidal Caring Ability Scale and the Suicide Attitudes Scale but no statistically significant differences in the Caring Stress Scale. That is, the suicide education program can promote the ability to care for people who are suicidal and can generate a positive attitude towards people who are suicidal from their caregivers (Sun, Chiang, Lin & Chen, 2014).

Pfeiffer et al. (2014) examined the effectiveness the telephone-based problem-solving intervention (PSI) for family caregivers of stroke survivors after the early post-stroke period. This was a randomized controlled trial. The including criteria of family caregivers were who provided care for at least 6 months and who experienced significant strain in their role. The PSI was composed of 2 home visits and 18 telephone calls delivered over a 3-month intensive intervention and a 9-month maintenance period. PSI and control groups received monthly information letters in addition to usual care. Primary caregiver outcomes were depressive symptoms (measure: Center for Epidemiologic Studies–Depression Scale) and sense of competence (measure: Sense of Competence Questionnaire). Their results indicated that caregivers of the PSI group showed significantly lower levels of depressive symptoms after 3 months and after 12 months, but no better sense of competence compared with the control group (Pfeiffer et al., 2014).

Northouse et al. (2013) examined (i) whether patient-caregiver dyads (i.e., pairs) randomly assigned to a brief or extensive dyadic intervention (the *FOCUS Program*) had better outcomes, quality of life (QOL), than dyads randomly assigned to usual care and (ii) whether patients' risk for distress and other factors moderated the effect of the brief or extensive program on outcomes. Advanced cancer patients and their caregivers ($N = 484$ dyads) were stratified by patients' baseline risk for distress (high versus low), cancer type (lung, colorectal, breast, or prostate), and research site and then randomly assigned to a brief (three-session) or extensive (six-session) intervention or control. The interventions offered dyads information and support.

Intermediary outcomes were appraisals (i.e., appraisal of illness/caregiving, uncertainty, and hopelessness) and resources (i.e., coping, interpersonal relationships, and self-efficacy). The primary outcome was QOL. The results indicated that there was a significant improvement in dyads' coping, self-efficacy, and social QOL and in caregivers' emotional QOL (Northouse et al., 2013).

MacNeil and Jaggers (2013) examined the effectiveness of the *Banking Positives intervention* among the family caregivers of patients with serious mental illness (SMI). The Banking Positives intervention uses elements of *cognitive therapy* to help family caregivers to generate positive emotions in coping situations. There were 10 family caregivers (7 female and 3 male) recruited in this study in the Alabama, USA. The results indicated that pre-test scores on the Family Burden Interview averaged 16.30, compared with 10.50 on the post-test measures ($t = 2.41$, $p = .040$).

Zarit Burden Interview from a mean 51.40 at pretest to 43.50 at posttest ($t = 2.69$, $p = .025$). Therefore, there were significant improvements of relieving family caregiver burden after intervention (MacNeil & Jaggers, 2013).

Sharif, Shaygan, and Mani (2012) examined the effectiveness of *family psycho-education* in reducing patients' symptoms and on family caregiver burden. Patients in the experimental group received antipsychotic drug treatment and a psycho-educational program was arranged for their caregivers. The psycho-educational program consisted of ten 90-min sessions held during five weeks (two sessions in each week). Each caregiver attended 10 sessions (in five weeks). Compared with the control group, the experimental group showed significantly reduced symptom severity and caregiver burden both immediately after intervention and one month later (Sharif, Shaygan & Mani, 2012).

Kolbrun Svavarsdottir and Olafia Sigurdardottir (2013) examined the effectiveness of a two-to-three session *family therapeutic conversation intervention* (FAM-TCI) for primary and partner caregivers of children and adolescents in active cancer treatment on perceived family support and on expressive family functioning. There were 19 parent caregivers (10 primary, 9 partner) of children in active cancer medical treatment. Their results indicated that primary caregivers perceived significantly higher family support after the intervention compared to before. Those caregivers also reported significantly higher expressive family functioning and significantly higher emotional communication after the intervention. (Kolbrun Svavarsdottir & Olafia Sigurdardottir, 2013).

Pahlavanzade, Khosravi, and Moeini (2014) examined the effectiveness of a *family need-based program* on the burden of care in caregivers of leukemia patients. Caregivers of the experimental group attended five training sessions. The data collection tool of this study was the *Zarit Burden Scale*. It was completed by members of both groups before, immediately after, and 1 month after the intervention. Their results indicated that during the study period, burden slowly decreased in the experimental group and increased in the control group. The mean burden score in the experimental group significantly decreased in comparison with the control group ($P < 0.001$) (Pahlavanzade, Khosravi & Moeini, 2014).

Ridge et al. (2014) examined the effectiveness of *Diabetes-Oriented Learning Family Intervention (DOLFIN)* for caregivers of young persons with Type 1 diabetes. Participants were caregivers of young persons aged 10-18 years with a diagnosis of Type 1 diabetes of more than 12 months' duration in two inner-city South London hospitals.

Caregivers were invited to attend six sessions of a *group workshop* where they received emotional support, diabetes education and were taught motivational interviewing techniques to support their child. Participants discussed a variety of themes in session, including the increasing difficulty of diabetes management as children grow older, parenting techniques for managing diabetes in the home and the emotional challenges of having a child with a chronic illness (Ridge et al., 2014).

Table 3. Factors influencing family caregiver burden (n = 8)

Authors	Design	Family Caregivers	Instrument	Findings
Chiou et al. (2009)	Descriptive, cross-sectional research design	301 family caregivers of incapable older people and home-care services Mean age: 50.9 ± 13.3 72.4% Female	Social Support Scale, Family APGAR (adaptation, partnership, growth, affection, resolve), and Caregiver Burden Scale	Caregiver burden was likely to be higher when the caregivers had lower levels of family function and social support.
Ducharme et al. (2014)	A mixed research design	32 family caregivers of dementia patients Mean age: 54.28 ± 10.58 75% Female	The Family Caregivers Support Agreement (FCSA) tool	Caregivers wished primarily: (1) to receive more information on available help and financial resources; (2) to have their relatives feel valued as persons and to offer them stimulating activities adjusted to their residual abilities; (3) to reduce stress stemming from their caregiver role assumed at an early age and to have the chance to enjoy more time for themselves; and (4) to receive help at the right time and for the help to be tailored to their situation of caregiver of a young person.
Tremont, Davis, and Bishop (2006)	Descriptive, cross-sectional research design	72 family caregivers of dementia patients at home Mean age: 64.36 ± 11.66 77% Female	Geriatric Depression Scale, Activities of Daily Living, Revised Memory and Behavior Problems Checklist, Dementia Knowledge Test, State-Trait Anxiety Inventory (State Form), Zarit Burden Interview, and The McMaster Family Assessment Device	Higher levels of caregiver burden were significantly associated with increased caregiver depression and anxiety, greater frequency of memory and behavior problems in the dementia patient, worse activities of daily living, and poorer family functioning.

Authors	Design	Family Caregivers	Instrument	Findings
Williams and Bakitas (2012)	Phenomenological research design, Thematic analysis	135 family caregivers Mean age: 52±16.2 years (range: 18-84 years) 66.7% Female	Open-ended in-person interviews, ex. ''Tell me about your experience of caring for [patient].'' Ex. ''I'd like to hear anything you want to tell me about caring for [patient].''	Four inter-related themes emerged: 1) becoming a caregiver; 2) new and altered relationships; 3) personal responses to caregiving and 4) antecedents and social context.
Yeh and Bull (2009)	Descriptive, cross-sectional research design	50 family caregivers of congestive heart failure Mean age: 60.3 ± 14.4 70% Female	JAREL Spiritual Well-Being Scale, Carers' Assessments of Managing Index, Symptom Questionnaire	Family caregivers' positive spiritual well-being and coping strategies were inversely related to their negative mental health.
Yeh and Bull (2012)	Descriptive, cross-sectional research design	50 family caregivers of congestive heart failure Mean age: 60.3 ± 14.4 70% Female	Index of ADL, JAREL Spiritual Well-being Scale, Carers' Assessments of Managing Index, Care Continuity Scale, Caregiver Reaction Assessment	The best predictors of family caregiver burden, using the resiliency model, were the older persons' activities of daily living dependence, family support, quality of relationship, care continuity, coping strategies and spiritual well-being.
Yeh and Chang (2012)	Descriptive, cross-sectional research design	200 family caregivers of hospitalized patients Mean age: 45.77 ± 12.82 64.5% Female	Index of ADL, Psychological well-being Scale, Knowledge of caregiving, Carergiver Reaction Assessment	Three factors were found to predict significantly greater impact on a family caregiver: (1) lower scores of caregiving knowledge, (2) increasing patient's activities of daily living dependency and (3) lack of family support.
Yeh, Wierenga, and Yuan (2009)	Descriptive, cross-sectional research design	91 family caregivers of hospitalized cancer patients Mean age: 46.65 ± 13.28 75.8% Female	Psychological Well-Being Scale, Carergiver Reaction Assessment	Psychological well-being, quality of caregiver-patient relationship, and family support accounted for 59% of the variance in caregivers' health.

Conclusion

Most of the interventional studies were effective in this review. Their interventions included education, providing information, and psychological well-being support. Most of their interventions were over than 2 hours and multiple times to follow up. Zarit Burden Interview has been used in many studies to measure family caregiver burden. In conclusion, these successful interventional studies were good examples to decrease family caregiver burden and improve family caregivers' quality of life.

References

Chiou, C. J., Chang, H. Y., Chen, I. P. & Wang, H. H. (2009). Social support and caregiving circumstances as predictors of caregiver burden in Taiwan. *Archives of Gerontology and Geriatrics, 48*(3), 419-424.

Ducharme, F., Kergoat, M. J., Coulombe, R., Lévesque, L., Antoine, P. & Pasquier, F. (2014). Unmet support needs of early-onset dementia family caregivers: a mixed-design study. *BMC Nursing, 13*(1), 1-20.

Etemadifar, S., Bahrami, M., Shahriari, M., Khosravi Farsani, A. (2014). The effectiveness of a supportive educative group intervention on family caregiver burden of patients with heart failure. *Iranian Journal of Nursing & Midwifery Research, 19*(3), 217-223.

Given, C. W., Given, B., Stommel, M., Collins, C., King, S. & Franklin, S., (1992). The caregiver reactions assessment (CRA) for caregivers to persons with chronic physical and mental impairments. *Research in Nursing & Health, 15*(4), 271-283.

Ridge, K., Thomas, S., Jackson, P., Pender, S., Heller, S., Treasure, J. & Ismail, K. (2014). Diabetes-Oriented Learning Family Intervention (DOLFIN): a feasibility study evaluating an intervention for carers of young persons with Type 1 diabetes. *Diabetic Medicine, 31*(1), 55-60.

Hudson, P., Trauer, T., Kelly, B., O'Connor, M., Thomas, K., Summers, M., Zordan, R. & White, V. (2013). Reducing the psychological distress of family caregivers of home-based palliative care patients: short-term effects from a randomised controlled trial. *Psycho-Oncology, 22*(9), 1987-1993.

Joling, K. J., Bosmans, J. E., van Marwijk, H. W. J., van der Horst, H. E., Scheltens, P., Vroomen, J. L. M. & van Hout, H. P. J. (2013). The cost-effectiveness of a family meetings intervention to prevent depression and anxiety in family caregivers of patients with dementia: a randomized trial. *Trials, 14*(1), 1-13.

Kolbrun Svavarsdottir, E. & Olafia Sigurdardottir, A. (2013). Benefits of a Brief Therapeutic Conversation Intervention for Families of Children and Adolescents in Active Cancer Treatment. *Oncology Nursing Forum, 40*(5), *E346-E357.*

MacNeil, G. & Jaggers, J. (2013). Banking Positives: A Strengths-Based Intervention for Long-Term Family Caregivers. *Best Practice in Mental Health, 9*(2), 102-113.

Moieni, M., Poorpooneh, Z. & Pahlavanzadeh, S. (2014). Investigating the effect of family-focused nursing intervention on caregiver burden of the family members of the patients undergoing coronary bypass surgery in Isfahan Shahid Chamran Hospital during 2012. *Iranian Journal of Nursing & Midwifery Research, 19*(2), 187-192.

Navidian, A., Pahlavanzadeh, S. & Yazdani, M. (2010). The effectiveness of family training on family caregivers of inpatients with mental disorders. *Iranian Journal of Psychiatry and Clinical Psychology, 16*(2), 99-106.

Northouse, L. L., Mood, D. W., Schafenacker, A., Kalemkerian, G., Zalupski, M., LoRusso, P., Hayes, D. F., Hussain, M., Ruckdeschel, J., Fendrick, A. M., Trask, P. C., Ronis, D. L. & Kershaw, T. (2013). Randomized clinical trial of a brief and extensive dyadic intervention for advanced cancer patients and their family caregivers. *Psycho-Oncology, 22*(3), 555-563.

Pahlavanzade, S., Khosravi, N. & Moeini, M. (2014). The effect of a family need-based program on burden of caregivers of leukemia patients in Isfahan in 2013-2014. *Iranian Journal of Nursing & Midwifery Research, 19*(6), 629-634.

Pfeiffer, K., Beische, D., Hautzinger, M., Berry, J. W., Wengert, J., Hoffrichter, R., Becker, C., van Schayck, R. & Elliott, T. R. (2014). Telephone-based problem-solving intervention for family caregivers of stroke survivors: A randomized controlled trial. *Journal of Consulting and Clinical Psychology, 82*(4), 628-643.

Sharif, F., Shaygan, M. & Mani, A. (2012). Effect of a psycho-educational intervention for family members on caregiver burdens and psychiatric symptoms in patients with schizophrenia in Shiraz, Iran. *BMC Psychiatry, 12*(48), 1-9.

Sigalet, E., Cheng, A., Donnon, T., Koot, D., Chatfield, J., Robinson, T., Catena, H., Grant, V. J. (2014). A simulation-based intervention teaching seizure management to caregivers: A randomized controlled pilot study. *Paediatrics & Child Health (1205-7088), 19* (7), 373-378.

Sun, F. K., Chiang, C. Y., Lin, Y. H. & Chen, T. B. (2014). Short-term effects of a suicide education intervention for family caregivers of people who are suicidal. *Journal of Clinical Nursing, 23*(1/2), 91-102.

Sun, F. K. & Long, A. (2008). A theory to guide families and carers of people who are at risk of suicide. *Journal of Clinical Nursing, 17*, 1939–1948.

Tremont, G., Davis, J. D. & Bishop, D. S. (2006). Unique contribution of family functioning in caregivers of patients with mild to moderate dementia. *Dementia & Geriatric Cognitive Disorders, 21* (3), 170-174.

Williams, A.-l. & Bakitas, M. (2012). Cancer Family Caregivers: A New Direction for Interventions. *Journal of Palliative Medicine, 15*(7), 775-783.

Yeh, P. M. & Bull, M. (2009). Influences of Spiritual Well-being and Coping on Family Caregiver Mental Health. *Research in Gerontological Nursing, 2*(3), 173-181.

Yeh, P. M. & Bull, M. (2012). Use of Resiliency Model of Family Stress, Adjustment, and Adaptation in Analysis of Family Caregiver Reaction among Families of Older People with Congestive Heart Failure. *International Journal of Older People Nursing*, 7(2), 117-126.

Yeh, P. M. & Chang, Y. M. (2012). Family Caregiver Reactions and Related Factors among Taiwanese with Hospitalized Relatives. *Journal of Advanced Nursing, 68*(10), 2195-2206.

Yeh, P. M., Wierenga, M. E. & Yuan, S. J. (2009). Influences of Psychological Well-being, Quality of Caregiver-Patient Relationship, and Family Support on the Health of Family Caregivers for Cancer Patients in Taiwan. *Asian Nursing Research, 3*(4), 1-13.

Zarit, S., Reever, K. & Bach-Peterson, J. (1980). Relatives of the impaired elderly: Correlates of feelings of burden. *Gerontologist, 20*(6), 649–655.

In: Caregivers
Editor: Adrienne Lloyd
ISBN: 978-1-63483-909-9

Chapter 2

QUALITY OF LIFE AND CAREGIVER BURDEN AMONG CAREGIVERS OF PATIENTS WITH CHRONIC LIVER DISEASE

Stephanie Y. Lee, MD, Matthew L. Bechtold, MD, M. Mazen Jamal, MD and Douglas L. Nguyen*, MD
Department of Medicine, UC Irvine School of Medicine,
Orange, CA, US

ABSTRACT

Chronic liver disease (CLD) and cirrhosis are currently the 12th leading cause of death in the United States [1]. Due to ongoing cost-containment efforts, there is an increased need for family-based care of chronically ill individuals. Debilitating symptoms of fatigue, pruritus, ascites, malnutrition, and encephalopathy are common manifestations of patients with CLD.

The presence of CLD at home has a significant impact on the primary caregivers and affects their overall quality of life. Several studies demonstrated a significantly lower mental health component on the quality of life assessment among caregivers of CLD patients.

However, only a minority of caregivers reported a formal clinical diagnosis for depression or anxiety, underscoring the fact that a significant number of caregivers may have undiagnosed clinical depression. Chronic depression and stress in the presence of inadequate resources and increasing patient dependency has been linked to decline in both physical and mental health status of patients and caregivers. While physicians are coached to "treat the whole patient," the future of longitudinal care for chronic diseases, including advanced liver disease, may require treating the person seated next to the patient as well.

* Corresponding Author: Douglas L. Nguyen MD, Assistant Clinical Professor of Medicine, Phone: 714-456-6745, Fax: 714-456-7753, Email: douglaln@uci.edu.

Introduction

In the United States, the impact of cirrhosis on the health care system has been increasing. While in 1990, cirrhosis was the 14th disease contributing to premature death, by 2010, it was the 8th leading contributor [2]. It is also a significant cause of disability among patients, ranking 16th amongst diseases contributing to disability-adjusted life-years [2]. Worldwide, cirrhosis is the 14th most common cause of death [3], leading to over 1 million deaths in 2010 [4].

While cirrhosis clearly leads to significant morbidity and mortality amongst patients, the burden of cirrhosis on the family unit, consisting of patients and their caregivers, is relatively unknown. By determining the most common physical and mental manifestations of caregiver burden, it may be possible to develop screening protocols and have ancillary resources available for caregivers to help relieve stressors and potentially improve patient outcomes. The liver disease-related factors that contribute the most to caregiver burden, such as those explored by previous studies, may help providers identify caregivers at high risk for burden-related problems. The diagnoses and specific complications that result from caregiver burden, including depression, anxiety, other mental illness, financial loss, and difficulties with personal relationships, also requires further study. Not only is it important to understand the burden of CLD on the family unit for the health of the caregivers, but the patient's adherence to medical therapy and transplant eligibility is dependent on the ability of the family to absorb these challenges as well.

The Need for Caregiving amongst Cirrhotic Patients

In 2012, Rakoski and colleagues found that in addition to requiring more healthcare services (hospitalizations, nursing home stays and physician visits) than age-matched control subjects, community-dwelling cirrhotic patients (that is, those residing at home rather than a nursing facility) require more caregiver hours [5]. Of those they studied, one-third of cirrhotic patients identified a caregiver, and less than 10% had formal, paid caregivers. Additionally, these patients reported over two times the informal caregiving hours compared with matched controls, leading to an approximate annual cost of $4,700 per person.

Socioeconomic Impact of Cirrhosis on Patients and Caregivers

Bajaj and colleagues studied the socioeconomic impact of cirrhosis on caregivers. Although caregivers of cirrhotic patients did not appear to have an increased financial burden compared with other caregivers based on the Perceived Caregiver Burden scale, it is important to note that there is a significant impact of cirrhosis on a patient's ability to work as 44% of patients had to stop working after being diagnosed with cirrhosis [6]. Furthermore, of the 56% of patients who were able to keep working, 53% of these patients had to decrease their hours at work [6]. Amongst caregivers of CLD patients, Nguyen and colleagues reported that as many as 48% of caregivers were actively working, either part-time or full-time. Eleven of 50 caregivers included (22%) reported having to stop working because of caregiving for the patients [7]. Miyazaki and colleagues reported that amongst caregivers of patients awaiting liver transplant, 59% had to give up or reduce their professional activities because of the demands associated with the caregiving role.

Physical Health of Caregivers of CLD Patients

Despite the fact that caregivers often have a personal history of chronic medical condition, caregivers of CLD patients experience limited quality-of-life from a physical health standpoint less frequently than caregivers of other patients. On the SF-36 Health Survey, CLD caregivers had a similar physical component score as the established US norm [7]. This is in contrast to other studies among caregivers of patients with advanced disease such as cancer and dementia [8-10]. The difference between caregivers of CLD patients and other chronic illnesses could be due to the fact that CLD patients are more likely to have an indolent course of illness compared to patients with advanced cancer who are more likely to have a more progressive disease course. Therefore, caring for liver patients may be less physically demanding than caring for patients with more rapid deterioration in physical health such as cancer and dementia.

Psychosocial Impact on Caregivers

Although the caregiver role can be associated with a sense of reward, including positive feelings, and gains felt from providing care for family [11], the role can also be associated with significant psychosocial burden. Miyazaki and colleagues reported that 25% of caregivers of patients awaiting liver transplant felt unprepared for this role. Common stressors amongst these caregivers include uncertainty about how to handle emergencies (reported by 42.6% of caregivers), dealing with mood swings of the patient (29.5% of caregivers), and concerns regarding patient adherence to treatment (11%) [12].

Compared with established National norms primary caregivers of liver patients scored lower on quality-of-life domains of limitation in role functioning due to emotional health, vitality, mental health and social functioning based on the Medical Outcome Study SF-36 Health Survey [7]. Overall, caregivers of patients with CLD have a significantly lower mental component score (MCS) at nearly one standard deviation below the reported National norm [7]. Surprisingly, though only 8 of 48 caregivers (16.7%) included in the analysis reported a formal clinical diagnosis for depression or anxiety, 23 participants (47.9%) had MCS < 42, a strong predictor of clinical depression [13-15]. Similarly, Bajaj and colleagues reported that while 17% of caregivers were being treated with antidepressants, 28% of caregivers had depression based on the Beck Depression Inventory (BDI; 18%, 5%, and 5% of caregivers with mild, moderate, and severe depression, respectively) [6]. Prevalence of depression may increase with disease severity, as Miyazaki and colleagues reported that amongst caregivers of liver transplant candidates, 75.4% had BDI scores suggestive of mild depression. This discrepancy between those with likely depression and those being treated for depression underscores the fact that many caregivers of cirrhotic patients may have undiagnosed clinical depression. Chronic depression and stress in the presence of inadequate resources and increasing patient dependency has been linked to decline in both physical and mental health status of patients and caregivers of other chronic disease conditions [12, 16-22].

PREDICTORS OF CAREGIVER BURDEN

Studies have used the Zarit Burden Interview to look for factors predictive of caregiver burden. This scale consists of 22 questions, rating 0-9 (9 – highest level of burden) and measures physical, emotional, and financial toll of providing care [23-25]. Cirrhosis impacts the family unit in terms of employment and finances [6]. Indeed, a lower household income, specifically less than $30,000, is a predictor of burden [6-7], and correlates with increased depressive symptoms, anxiety levels, and subjective burden amongst caregivers [26]. Additionally, having one or more dependents at home other than the patients are also predictors of caregiver burden [7, 26].

Patients who require more than 2 hospitalizations related to liver disease over 12 months also place a toll on the caregiver [7]. Increased rates of hospitalization due to severely decompensated liver disease and comorbidities can increase the challenge of caregiving. This underscores the need to optimize management in patients with advanced liver disease to prevent complications for both the patient and caregiver's well-being.

In terms of patient-specific predictors of caregiver burden, a history of hepatic encephalopathy in the patient correlates with burden [6-7] as this can impact a caregiver's schedule and lead to a sense of entrapment [6]. It is unclear whether MELD score is predictive of caregiver burden. While some studies suggest that a higher MELD score is associated with greater caregiver burden [6, 12], others did not detect a difference in caregiver burden when using a MELD threshold of 18 [7]. In terms of the etiology of cirrhosis, while previous studies have demonstrated that alcoholic cirrhosis led to increased caregiver burden compared to other causes of cirrhosis [14], it appears that active alcohol use in the patient is also strongly associated with an increased burden [7].

ADDRESSING CAREGIVER BURDEN

Previous studies have demonstrated that in other chronic diseases, social support groups for caregivers may also reduce caregiver burden and burnout [27-28]. As an example, Han and colleagues found that caregivers of dementia patients experience reduced psychological burden when offered positive social interactions (in which others are available for fun activities with the caregiver) and affectionate support (involving expressions of love and affection). Tangible support (material aid or behavioral assistance) leads to a reduction in non-psychological burden in this group [28]. Lopez-Hartmann and colleagues reviewed various support services for caregivers of elderly individuals within the community and found inconsistent results. This suggests that there may not be a "best caregiver support" for caregivers of this population [27].

While it is possible that there may not be a support system that is beneficial to all caregivers of CLD patients, development of a multidisciplinary treatment team for CLD patients has shown some promise. Specifically, a specialized multidisciplinary care management team to manage complications related to CLD such as depression, ascites, malnutrition, and variceal bleeding in the outpatient setting may reduce caregiver burden and patient hospitalization. Morando et al. demonstrated that such a multidisciplinary approach for outpatient management of cirrhotics can reduce 12-month mortality. Their approach included an integrated team including consultant hepatologists, dedicated nurses and physicians in training that followed the patient as needed based on laboratory results and procedures performed, and continued to follow the patient in the hospital setting. This approach was compared to standard care in which a primary physician is mainly responsible for the management of cirrhotic patients with a specialist who followed as needed, with or without laboratory or procedure data, and in which the specialist following the patient during hospitalization could be different from the specialist caring for the patient in the outpatient setting. Compared with standard care, the multidisciplinary approach was associated with a significantly lower 12-month mortality (23.1% compared with 45.4% in the standard care group). Additionally 30-day readmission rate was lower for patients receiving multidisciplinary care (15.4% in the multidisciplinary group versus 42.4% in the standard care group). Furthermore, global cost attributable to management per month of life was lower for those receiving multidisciplinary care [29]. Since this approach has the potential to reduce hospitalizations and cost, by extension, it may also prove to be helpful at reducing caregiver burden.

Conclusion

CLD has a profound impact on both the patient and family unit. In treating patients with CLD, it is important that providers recognize signs of caregiver burden, particularly in light of the fact that studies suggest that many CLD caregivers may have undiagnosed clinical depression. When healthcare providers encounter CLD patients with lower household income, continued alcohol use, a history of hepatic encephalopathy, or a history of frequent hospitalizations, they should pay particular attention not only to the patient, but the caregiver as well, as these factors are associated with increased caregiver burden. In addition to addressing caregiver burden directly, multidisciplinary approaches to managing patients with CLD have shown promise at improving outcomes of both patients and caregivers alike.

References

[1] Murphy, SL, J Xu, and KD Kochanek. "Deaths: final data for 2010." *Natl. Vital. Stat. Rep.* 61, no. 1-117 (2013).

[2] US Burden of Disease Collaborators. "The state of US health, 1990-2010: burden of diseases, injuries, and risk factors." *JAMA* 310 (2013): 591-608.

[3] Tsochatzis, EA, J Bosch, and AK Burroughs. "Liver cirrhosis." *Lancet* 383 (2014): 1749-1761.

[4] Lozano, R, M Naghavi, K Foreman, and et al. "Global and regional mortality from 235 causes of death for 20 age groups in 1990 and 2010: a systematic analysis for the Global Burden of Disease Study 2010." *Lancet* 380 (2012): 2095-2128.
[5] Rakoski, MO, et al. "Burden of cirrhosis on older Americans and their families: analysis of the health and retirement study." *Hepatology* 55, no. 1 (January 2012): 184-191.
[6] Bajaj, JS, JB Wade, DP Gibson, and et al. "The multi-dimensional burden of cirrhosis and hepatic encephalopathy on patients and caregivers." *Am. J. Gastro* 106, no. 9 (2011): 1646-53.
[7] Nguyen, DL, D Chao, G Ma, and T Morgan. "Quality of life and factors predictive of burden among primary caregivers of chronic liver disease patients." *Annals of Gastroenterology* 28 (2015): 124-129.
[8] Butow, PN, MA Price, ML Bell, and et al. "Caring for women with ovarian cancer in the last year of life: a longitudinal study of caregiver quality of life, distress and unmet needs." *Gynecol. Oncol.* 132 (2014): 690-697.
[9] Li, TC, YD Lee, CC Lin, and RL Amidon. "Quality of life of primary caregivers of elderly with cerebrovascular disease or diabetes hospitalized for acute care: assessment of well-being and functioning using the SF-36 health questionnaire." *Qual. Life Res.* 13 (2004): 1081-1088.
[10] Tan, SB, AF Williams, ME Morris, and EK Tan. "Health-related quality of life of caregivers of people with Parkinson's disease in Singapore." *Proc. Singapore Healthc* 19 (2010): 297-302.
[11] Picot, S. "Rewards, costs and coping of African American caregivers." *Nursing Research* 44, no. 3 (1995): 147-152.
[12] Miyazaki, ET, R Dos Santos, MC Miyazaki, and et al. "Patients on the waiting list for liver transplantation: caregiver burden and stress." *Liver Transpl.* 16 (2010): 1164-1168.
[13] Silveira, E, C Taft, V Sundh, M Waern, S Palsson, and B Steen. "Performance of the SF-36 health survey in screening for depressive and anxiety disorders in an elderly female Swedish population." *Qual. Life Res.* 14 (2005): 1263-1274.
[14] Elliott, TE, CM Renier, and JA Palcher. "Chronic pain, depression, and quality of life: correlations and predictive value of the SF-36." *Pain Med.* 4 (2003): 331-339.
[15] Ware, JE, KK Snow, M Kosinski, and et al. *SF-36 Health Survey Manual and Interpretation Guide.* Boston, MA: New England Medical Center, The Health Institute, 1993.
[16] Pearlin, LI, JT Mullan, SJ Semple, and MM Skaff. "Caregiving and the stress process: an overview of concepts and their measures." *Gerontologist* 30 (1990): 583-594.
[17] Bolkhir, A, MM Loiselle, DM Evon, and PH Hayashi. "Depression in primary caregivers of patients listed for liver or kidney transplantation." *Prog. Transplant.* 17 (2007): 193-198.
[18] Goetzinger, AM, JA Blumenthal, CV O'Hayer, and et al. "Stress and coping in caregivers of patients awaiting solid organ transplantation." *Clin. Transplant* 26 (2012): 97-104.
[19] Yikilkan, H, C Aypak, and S Gorpelioglu. "Depression, anxiety and quality of life in caregivers of long-term home care patients." *Arch. Psychiatr Nurs.* 28 (2014): 193-196.

[20] Grunfeld, E, D Coyle, T Whelan, and et al. "Family caregiver burden: results of a longitudinal study of breast cancer patients and their principle caregivers." *CMAJ* 170 (2004): 1795-1801.

[21] Andrews, SC. "Caregiver burden and symptom distress in people with cancer receiving hospice care." *Oncol. Nurs. Forum* 28 (2001): 1469-1474.

[22] Kozachik, SL, CW Given, BA Given, and et al. "Improving depressive symptoms among caregivers of patients with cancer: results of a randomized clinical trial." *Oncol. Nurs. Forum* 28 (2001): 1149-1157.

[23] Gort, AM, M Mingot, X Gomez, and et al. "Use of the Zarit scale for assessing caregiver burden and collapse in caregiving at home in dementias." *Int. J. Geriatr Psychiatry* 22 (2007): 957-962.

[24] Ballesteros, J, B Santos, E Gonzalez-Fraile, P Munoz-Hermoso, AI Dominguez-Panchon, and M Martin-Carrasco. "Unidimensional 12-item Zarit Caregiver Burden Interview for the assessment of dementia caregivers' burden obtained by item response theory." *Value Health* 15 (2012): 1141-1147.

[25] Seng, BK, N Luo, WY Ng, and et al. "Validity and reliably of the Zarit Burden Interview in assessing caregiving burden." *Ann. Acad. Med. Singapore* 39 (2010): 758-763.

[26] Bolden, L, and MN Wicks. "Predictors of mental health, subjective burden, and rewards in family caregivers of patients with chronic liver disease." *Arch. Psychiatr. Nurs.* 24 (2010): 89-103.

[27] Lopez-Hartmann, M, J Wens, V Verhoeven, and R Remmen. "The effect of caregiver support interventions for informal caregivers of community-dwelling frail elderly: a systematic review." *Int. J. Integr. Care* 12 (2012): e133.

[28] Han, JW, H Jeong, JY Park, and et al. "Effects of social supports on burden in caregivers of people with dementia." *Int. Psychogeriatr*, 2014: 1-10.

[29] Morando, F, G Maresio, S Piano, and et al. "How to improve care in outpatients with cirrhosis and ascites: a new model of care coordination by consultant hepatologists." *J. Hepatol.* 59 (2013): 257-264.

In: Caregivers
Editor: Adrienne Lloyd
ISBN: 978-1-63483-909-9

Chapter 3

EPILEPSY AND SELF ESTEEM: PATHWAYS TO LESSENING CAREGIVER BURDEN

Adebayo David Oluwole*, PhD
Department of Guidance & Counselling
University of Ibadan, Nigeria

ABSTRACT

The burden of caring for the epileptics places a toll on stakeholders of epilepsy management. It is hence very essential to understand the cross cultural psychology of epilepsy, origin of epilepsy, prevalence of epilepsy worldwide and the Nigerian perspective on epilepsy pathology and management of epileptics' self esteem.

Epilepsy is not yet clearly understood and there is no known cure. Because of this, and the historical context, fear of the disorder is widespread. At one time the disorder was thought to be caused by the possession of a person by the devil and even today, myths, misunderstandings and social stigma still exist. As a result, the patient may fear rejection by peers and employers and decidedly refuse to disclose the health problem even though it would be wiser to do so.

The epilepsies are characterized by sudden seizure caused by a disruption of activity in the brain cells. While in some cases the cause of epilepsy can be determined (usually a head injury or brain tumor), generally the origin of the seizure is unknown.

It is notable that upping the self esteem of the epileptics should be paramount in psychotherapeutic management of epilepsy.

Keywords: epilepsy, self esteem, caregiver burden, Nigeria

ORIGIN OF EPILEPSY

Epilepsy is a global health problem, which has attracted the attention of many researchers. Epilepsy was one of the first brain disorders to be described. It was mentioned in

* +2348034105253, daoluwoledr@gmail.com.

ancient Babylon more than 3,000 years ago. Epilepsy is an ancient disease, Hippocrates (460-377 BC) defined it as a chronic functional (having no organic base) disease, characterized by fits or attacks in which there is loss of consciousness with a succession of tonic (increased muscle tone) and clonic (involuntary muscular contractions) convulsion. These attitudes from the society made epileptics to see themselves as people separated from others which led to low self-esteem.

It has been recognized from time immemorial that certain people are liable to suffer from fits and this condition has been called epilepsy or the "falling sickness" Hippocrates (460-477) used the word epilepsy to indicate something with "seized" upon the patient. For many centuries such seizures were thought to be due to possession by demons or evil spirits. Epileptics were therefore regarded with superstitious fear and even today this attitude persists to some extent and often increases the difficulties within the life of the patient (Ackner, 2005). In ancient Greece, epilepsy was referred to as the "sacred disease," a sign of honor given by the gods. In Tanzania to this day as with other parts of Africa, epilepsy is associated with possession of evil spirits, witchcraft, or poisoning and is believed by many to be contagious (Wikipedia, 2009, Jilek-all, 1999). In Cameroon, it is believed that people with epilepsy are inhabited by the devil. This does not mean that they are seen as evil, but that evil evades them and causes them to convulse from time to time. Epilepsy is often considered as a punishment from unknown dark forces as believed by the Indonesians. In Uganda, epilepsy is thought to be contagious and so people with epilepsy are not allowed to join the communal food pot for fear of others contracting epilepsy through that person's saliva (Dada (1970); Osuntokun and Odeku (1970) and Osuntokun (1979) asserted that Nigerians believe that epilepsy is infectious, a dreadful disease inflicted on victims by the devil, and transmitted from one patient to another via saliva. Epilepsy is described as a "social disgrace," as an illness that afflict only the possessed and the worse disaster that can befall anyone (Osunton and Odeku, 1970).

The strange behaviour caused by some seizures has contributed through the ages to many superstitious and prejudices (National Institute of Neurological Disorders and Stroke, 2010). Gelder, Harrison and Cowe (2006) wrote that in most parts of the world epilepsy is still believed to be caused by evil spirits. It is one of the oldest diseases known to man. In the past, epilepsy was associated with religious experiences and even with demonic possession. The ailment was viewed as being divine in origin and was called "the sacred disease" because it was believed that a person with epilepsy was "seized" by gods (Macleod & Austin, 2003). Watson and Royle (2002) reported that many famous and productive people throughout history were subject to seizures. Notable among them are Julius Caesar, William Pitt, Lord Byron, Charles Dickens, Martin Luther, Vincent Van Gogh, Ludwig Van, Beethoven, George Handel, Peter Ilyich Tchaikovsky, Alfred Nobel and Dostoyevsky. The Holy Bible also gave account of epileptic seizures in Mark 9:17-27. Modern investigators believe that epilepsy is caused by disease germs and this agrees with Hippocrates (460_477 BC) who had a debunked belief that those afflicted with epilepsy were possessed by gods or goddesses. He proposed that epilepsy was a brain disease caused by the blockage` of phlegm of the air-carrying vessels to the brain which could be treated with medicine and diet (The Commission for the Control of Epilepsy and its Consequences, 1997).

Epilepsy is a common chronic neurological disorder that is characterized by recurrent unprovoked seizures (Blume and others, 2001). These seizures are transient signs and/or symptoms of abnormal, excessive or hyper-synchronous neurological activity in the brain,

(Fisher, Van Emde Boas, Brume, Elger, Genton, Lee and Engel, 2005). Epilepsy is not a single disorder, but rather as syndromic with vastly divergent symptoms but all involving episodic abnormal electrical activity in the brainEpileptic fit is generally a sign of nervous system disease (e.g., brain tumour) or it may be a sign of systematic or metabolic derangement (Gelder, Harrison and Cowe, 2006). Systemic condition in which seizure most commonly occur include general hypoglycemia, hypocalcaemia (tetany) renal in sufficiency (uraemia) hypoxia, high fever especially in children, toxaemia of pregnancy and chemical poisoning (e.g., alcohol, strychime, amphetamine, lead and inhalation of insecticide). During adolescence and adulthood, the causes of epilepsy are more likely to be secondary to any Central Nervous System (CNS) lesion. These include stress, trauma, CNS infections, brain tumors, illicit drug use and alcohol withdrawal. In older adults cerebrovascular disease (CVS) is a very common cause. Other causes are CNS tumors, head injury (trauma) and other degenerative diseases that are common in older group, such as dementia (Frucht, Quigg, Schwaner & Fountain, 2000).

Epilepsy is more likely to occur in young children, or people over the age of 65 years, however, it can occur at any time in life (The National Society for Epilepsy, 2009). As a consequence of brain surgery, epileptic seizures may occur in recovering patients. Clients may be prone to seizures due to permanent or temporary medical conditions such as drug reactions or extreme fever (Berman, Snyder, Kozier and Erb, 2008). However, about 50% of seizures/ epileptic fits have no known cause (Cross, 2004). A family history of epilepsy may suggest a genetic cause when seizure disorders develop in individuals aged 5 to 25 years (Osuntokun, 1978).

The disorder characterized by recurring seizures and commonly referred to as epilepsy represents one of the most common neurological disorder affecting individuals irrespective of geographical location, gender and race (Walsh, 2005). About one person has a seizure of some type during life. In the population at large, about one in 200 has epilepsy (Watson &Royle, 2002). Most new-onset of epilepsy is idiopathic and occurs before the age of 20 years. Other frequent causes include trauma, in the third and fourth decades, neoplasms in the fifth and sixth decades, and cerebrovascular disease in the elderly. Although some complex partial seizures originate from frontal or temporal neo cortex and other areas, at least two thirds of complex partial seizures and generalized tonic-clonic seizures originate from the mediobasal temporal limbic structures (hippocampus, amygdale, and parahippocampalgyrus), (Mendel, 1995).

A diagnosis of epilepsy is made when seizures occurs regularly and not in a single episode. A diagnosis of epilepsy is clinical and is based on eye witness account. It also rest largely on the history of the attack given by the patient. The information gives a clue to the location of the epileptogenic focus in the brain. The nature of the seizure usually indicates the type of treatment that is required. In addition to providing data about the seizure, the management care is directed at preventing injury and supporting the patient (Smeltzer& Bare, 2000). It is also made based on the medical history, electrocardiogram (ECG) brain scanning and magneto encephalography to discover aetiology for the epilepsy, discover the affected brain region, or classify the epileptic syndrome.

According to the International Classification System (1989), epilepsies and epileptic syndromes are classified into three main categories; (1) Localization- related, (2) Generalized, and (3) Undetermined. Epilepsies within category 1 are classified as idiopathic, symptomatic or cryptogenic cases, whereas those within category 2 are classified as idiopathic, cryptogenic/symptomatic and 3 symptomatic cases. Hoie (2007) asserted that in idiopathic epilepsies no underlying cause can be found to explain the seizures and the onset is frequently in childhood. Symptomatic epilepsies may occur at any age and mental retardation can be present. The etiology is known in such cases. In cryptogenic cases, the cause is unclear or hidden, but it is presumed that the epilepsy is symptomatic; example of this is childhood absence epilepsy, juvenile myoclonic epilepsy, infantile spasms etc.

In clinical practice epilepsies are also frequently divided into two main categories those with remote symptomatic etiology (known causes and those without such etiology (unknown causes). It classified seizures as grand and petit mal. Whereas grand mal was used to describe a generalized tonic-clonic convulsion, petit-mal was used to name any seizure that was not a convulsion. Hoie (2007) states that generalized tonic-colonic seizures (grand mal) start with tonic phase evolving to a clonic phase, typical absences (petit-mal) start and cease suddenly, whereas a typical absences have a slower start and termination and may be accompanied by movements. Gelder, Harrison & Cowen (2006) wrote about status epilepticus and noted that it is a succession of grand mal and stressed that it is a medical emergency which must be treated vigorously or the patient may die or his brain may be damaged.

CONCEPT OF EPILEPSY

Epilepsy refers to disorder of the brain characterized by recurrence of unpredictable interruptions of the of the normal brain function called epileptic seizures (Fisher, Van Emde Boas, Brume, Elger, Genton, Lee and Engel, (2005); World Health Organization (WHO, 2012). Epilepsy is one of the most common of the serious neurological disorders (Hirtz, Thurman, Gwinn-Hardy, Mohammed, Chandhuri, Zalutsky, 2007). About 3% of people will be diagnosed with epilepsy at some time in their lives (Hausa and Kurland, 1975). Epilepsy is a “hidden” or “invisible” disability, as no symptoms are apparent except during a seizure. Hills (2007) wrote that it often has no apparent cause which results in a fear of the unknown. Consequently it is easier to deny, resulting in poor compliance with treatment and a refusal to alter lifestyle. Being ‘hidden’ makes it more difficult for others wishing to interact, and concealment makes it difficult to find other people with epilepsy for support. Being ‘hidden’ may lead to accusations of hypochondria and misbehaviour as well as erroneous self-perception Hill emphasized.

Mood disorder, predominantly anxiety and depression, occur frequently in people with epilepsy. Pilo (1993) wrote that a number of factors have been linked to the pathogenesis of depression including patients fears, social stigma and adverse life events. Bhatia (2010) observed impulsive – irritable behaviour among epileptic patients that is characterized occasionally by abusiveness and displays of temper, which occurs without provocation or seems out of proportion to any precipitating stimulus. No seizure discharges occurs during this behaviour and events are fully recalled. Barraclough (1982) found that the risk of suicide was five times greater than that of general population and self-poisoning with barbiturates was the most common mode of suicide. Although epilepsy is a symptom of an illness, many caregivers thought it has a psychiatric origin and discriminate people with epilepsy. This could bring about social and psychological isolation leading to low self-esteem of the epileptic patients. By learning how to effectively deal with these problems, epileptic patients should learn to adhere to their medical and psychological treatment and control their behaviour pattern so that they can live happier and more productive lives.

Epilepsy affects 50 million people worldwide and more than 2.7 million people in the United States; half of all patients are children. Especially in its intractable forms, also called refractory epilepsy, the disorder and the side effects of epilepsy medications can cause problems in learning, memory and behaviour, and inability alter development (Devinsky, 2008). Devinsky asserts that despite the number of people with epilepsy, the disorder affects more Americans than do Parkinson's disease, multiple sclerosis and Lou Gebrig's disease combined; it still carries a stigma that dates to ancient civilization. The feeling from many caregivers, is that many patients, doctors and families say the stigma hampers care, public recognition and the ability to raise money for research. Epilepsy carry a lot worse stigma than a cancer, or an Human Immunodeficiency Virus (HIV).

Epilepsy is a sudden onset of excessive electrical discharge in one more areas of the brain; it can develop at any time during the person's life and occur at any time. According to Santrock (2003), epileptic seizures are the result of electrical "brainstorms" that flash uncontrollably, from one side of the brain to the other. Nerve cells on one side become more overactive and stimulate other activity in nerve cells on the other side. The excessive stimulation produces a seizure in which the individual loses consciousness and goes into convulsions. In severe cases, seizures can occur numerous times during the day (Walsh, 2005).

There are two main classification of epilepsy, partial and generalized. Partial seizures also called focal epilepsy involves discharges from one area of the brain and generalized epilepsy (seizures) that affect the whole brain (Berman, Snyder, Kozier and Erb 2008). Each of these seizures categories includes different types of seizures, depending on the characteristic of the seizure activity, for example loss of consciousness versus no impairment to consciousness. During partial seizure, the person can experience a range of strange or unusual sensations including sudden jerky movements of one body part, distortion in hearing or seeing, stomach discomfort, or a sudden sense of fear but consciousness is not impaired (Barry, 1982). Generalized seizure (formerly known as grand mal) is a generalized convulsion involving two phases. In the tonic phase, the individual loses consciousness, and falls and the body becomes rigid. In the clonic period, the body extremities jerk and twitch and the muscles also. This causes frost in the mouth mixed with blood, in continence of urine also occurs and it gradually phases out and the patient goes into deep sleep for minutes or hours. Watson and Royle (2002) postulate that Complex partial seizures (formerly psychomotor) are characterized by a complicated motor act involving impaired consciousness. During the seizure the patient appears dazed and confused, purposeless behaviours such as random walking, numbing, head turning or pulling at clothing may be observed (Ackner, 2005). Generalized absence seizures (formerly petit-mal) are characterized by 5 to 15 second lapses in consciousness. During this time the patient appears to be staring into space and the eyes may roll upwards and there will be a break in whatever the person was doing at that particular time (discussing with other people). Absences are not preceded by aura and activity can be resumed immediately afterwards (Watson and Royle, 2002). When seizure occurs frequently, a status epileptic ensures and full recovery of the brain function does not occur. This calls for medical emergency to revive the patient.

There are two broad types of seizures: partial seizure, which start in only a portion of the brain, and generalized seizures, which involve the entire brain Alloy, et al., (1999) asserts that the most common form of a complex partial seizure Interrupts cognitive functioning for up to several minutes. Between seizures, epileptics often complain of poor memories, though the disease can interfere with concentration and learning, many epileptics are treated with drugs which suppress seizures. If the drug treatment is unsuccessful, surgery can sometimes be performed to control the seizures. If seizures are not controlled, cognitive impairment and stigma constitutes and low self-esteem persists.

There are several experimental models that have been developed to study the mechanism of epilepsy. One of this is the evidence of disturbance in the excitory and inhibitory synapses impinging on the epileptic neuron (Solomon et al., 1983: Gelder et al., 2006). There is also indication of different degrees of epileptic neurons within the epileptic focus. In the normal brain, certain stability exists, the ability to suppress abnormal neural activity may be impaired or lost, or there may be increased excitation within the neurons Watson &Royle, (2002) and Walsh (2005) wrote that abnormal activity may occur in a small group of neurons and remain relatively localized or may spread to involve extensive areas of the neurons. According to Wyler and Ward, (1980) several epileptic nerve cells can stimulate the next level of epileptic nerve cells and thereby generate a seizure by recruiting the adjacent neurons. Researcher's has it that several chemical and structural alternations have been observed, both in within the epileptic focus and outside it, and they have provided evidence of possible mechanisms for epileptic activity. One of this is the loss of inhibitory neurons (usually from hypoxia) in the cerebellum, neocortex, and certain other structures in the cerebrum, which lead to seizure in many experimental situations (Meldrum, 1982).

Another alteration according to Loeser and Howe, (1980) is the loss of spines on the dendrites of neurons in the epileptic focus, which may be the reason for their hypersensitivity. It is common to see proliferation of fibrous astrocutes (glial scarring) in the epileptic focus, although the exact role this may play in generating seizure is not clear (Ozuna, 1982, Meldrum, 1982, 2008). Alteration in enzymes and neurotransmitter substances within the brain may also play a part in epileptic activity (Meldrum, 2002). Epilepsy may develop because of an abnormality in the brain wiring, an imbalance of nerve signaling chemicals called neurotransmitters, or some combination of these factors. Researchers believe that people with epilepsy have an abnormally high level of excitatory neurotransmitters that increases neuronal activity while others have abnormally low level of inhibitory neurotransmitters that decrease neural activity in the brain. Either situation can result in too much neuronal activity and causes epilepsy. One of the most –studied neurotransmitters that plays a role in epilepsy is GABA, or gamma – aminobutyric acid, which is an inhibitory neurotransmitters (National Institute of Neurological Disorders and Stroke, 2010).

Research has shown that the cell membrane that surrounds each neuron plays an important role in epilepsy. Cell membranes are crucial for a neuron to generate electrical impulses (how molecules move in and out of membranes and how the cell nourishes and repairs the membrane). A disruption in any of these processes may lead to epilepsy. National Institute of Neurological Disorders and Stroke (2010) wrote that studies in animals have shown that because the brain continually adapts to changes in stimuli, a small change in neuronal activity, if repeated, may eventually lead to full blown epilepsy.

In the 1800s, it was noted by Jackson that epileptic seizures begin in isolated parts of the body such as the thumb and from there spread to neighboring regions perhaps the arm and then to the rest of the body. He hypothesized that there were areas in cerebral cortex that controlled isolated movements and that the areas that were adjacent in the brain were anatomically adjacent as well. Therefore, a seizure began in one area and spread to the rest of the cortex. The body's movements are mapped out on this band giving rise to the spreading fashion that Jackson described during seizures Hausa (1955). Experimental work has demonstrated that repeated or prolonged seizures (status epilepticus) cause hippocampal sclerosis, presumably through excessive activation of excitatory glutamate receptors, which results in excitotoxicity. Removal of sclerotic hippocampus leads to dramatic improvement or even a cure of the epileptic condition in humans, which suggests that the sclerotic hippocampus somehow causes the epilepsy. In the absence of hypoxia though, it seems equally plausible that intense seizures can cause hippocampal sclerosis, which then can cause epilepsy.

Other factors that can provoke or increase the frequency of seizures in epileptic patients include Lack of sleep, Menstruation, Stress, Consumption of Alcohol, especially binge drinking which is especially bad for the people with epilepsy. Infections can increase the frequency of seizures and drugs such as tricyclic antidepressants, high doses of penicillin, or sudden withdrawal from other drugs (Ackner 2005).

Prevalence of Epilepsy Worldwide

Incidence and prevalence studies of epilepsy have been reported by various researchers from all over the world with different views. Bhatia (2010) opined that between 0.2 and 0.3 percent of the world population is affected by epileptic disorders. It usually starts in childhood and is common in all age groups and equally prevalent in both sexes. He asserted that prevalence rates of idiopathic epilepsy in the general population ranging from 2 – 20/1000 population. The incidence of epilepsy according to National Institutes of Health (2008) is about 1 in 200 people around the world and in the United States, there are close to one million people with epilepsy. The annual incidence rate of epilepsy is around 35-50 per 100,000 populations and the prevalent rate of epilepsy is 5 per 1,000 of the population Hauser and Kurland (1975) and Pond (1981). Shorvan and Farmer (1988) had incidence rates of 20-70/100,000 in the general population (range 1.5 -30/1000).

The incidence of epilepsy in Britain is about 1 in every 200 of the population, given a total figure of up to 200,000, about 80 percent of these live normal lives with a minimum of inconveniences. The prevalent rate in general population is 0.5 in England according to Trethowan (2001). Between 0.5% and 2% of the population or from 1 million to 4 million people in the United States of America have epilepsy. The outset of epilepsy occurs before the age of 20 years in 80% of cases (Ozuna, 1983). Accurate figures of the prevalence of epilepsy are difficult to obtain for two reasons. The first is variability in making a diagnosis of epilepsy in people who have recurring seizures from fibrile illness, recurring electrolyte imbalance, multiple infectious processes or brain tumors, to name a few. An example of this is the person who at one time had seizures due to a brain tumor but no longer has them since the tumor was removed. The second reason is that for wide variety of reasons many persons with epilepsy do not report their seizures. They may wish to avoid the social stigma, to maintain their driver's license, to avoid job discrimination, or simply to maintain privacy. Incidence varies considerably with age, rates are greatest in early childhood, reaching a plateau in early adult life, and risen again in elderly people. Prevalence rates show a similar but less pronounced age-nested pattern (Shorvan and Farmer, 1988; Olley, 1997). Incidence rates of epilepsy in Nigeria were reported by Osuntokun, Adeuja, Nottidge and Bademosi (1987) at a low prevalence rate of 5.3 per 1,000. In a study from Igbo-Ora. Dada (1970) estimated prevalence rate of 13 per 1,000 in Lagos State.

THE NIGERIAN PERSPECTIVE ON EPILEPSY PATHOLOGY

Epilepsy is a dreaded disease among Nigerians and most ethnic groups have names for it. The Ikwerres in Rivers state call it "Odakpui," among the Ibos "Akwukwu," among the Yorubas "Warapa," the Benis call it "Owa," the Urhobos "Wenwen" and the Efiks "Ndisi." The patients are called by these names which are pertained to the disease. This has caused emotional distress to those afflicted especially when it occurs frequently, and in the presence of those who think it is contagious thereby stigmatizing, the sufferers (Awaretefe, Longe&Awaretefe, 1985). People who witnessed seizures are frequently frightened and withdrawn from the patients and misinterpret the behaviour as having a psychiatric origin (Lovely and Ozuna, 1982; Russell, 1982; Ozuna, 1986). This in turn causes the epileptic patients to withdraw from the society and creates loss of self-esteem, and inability to cope. Some caregivers of persons with epilepsy may not allow their epileptic children to attend school in order to avoid bringing shame to the family. The epileptic patients may also be expelled by school authorities for fear of infecting others with the disease, school may not want to include students with epilepsy on field trips if they are admitted and peers may not invite them for sleep overs. Bergquist (2007) wrote that it is frightening to see a child's seizure, and people may become frightened. In Nigeria, many caregivers still believe that epilepsy is contagious and as adults, they have difficulties in finding or retaining a job and often meet with active discrimination when they seek employment. The epileptics have difficulties in keeping and making friends, in getting married, and in retaining their spouse (Osuntokun, 1979). People prefer a cured psychotic patient to an epileptic, which indicate general negative attitude toward epileptic patients than towards cured psychotic patients, according to one study in Benin Nigeria by Awaretefe, Longe and Awaretefe (1985). The belief of caregivers as regards the cause of epilepsy among Nigerians determines the kind of treatment given to cure it. Traditionally, these patients are treated with herbs and incantations. Among the Yorubas, lizard is believed to be inhibiting the brain of sufferers. Herbalists usually hypnotize the victims through incantations and the lizard is vomited to get healed. The Ibos and Efiks use both herbs and incantations to cure epilepsy and the patients normally stay with the healers for days or months depending on the severity of the illness. The overall treatment which is equally shrouded in mystery and sacrifices are employed in all cases. Meanwhile there are two types of epilepsy, the first type, the Yoruba calls it *Warapa,* causes foaming in the mouth. The second type, Yoruba calls *Ogun-Oru,* does not foam. In Igbo language it is called *Atakuku* or *Akuku*, in Hausa it is called *Farfadida*. When it attacks it leaves the victim partially helpless and the body becomes weak.

SELF ESTEEM, STIGMATISATION AND EPILEPSY

Epilepsy is known as a stigmatizing condition as people with epilepsy sometimes cannot conform to usual social norms as a result of the unpredictable nature of seizures; consequently, society may fear dealing with someone who is having an epileptic seizure (Jocoby, et al., 2005, Ablon, 2002, and Scamler and Hopkins, 1990). From the patient's point of view, the diagnosis of epilepsy challenges self-perception, and causes concern about ability to function in normal social roles, such as getting a job or having a family. (Scambler and Hopkins, 1990). They assert that the perception of epilepsy is often negative, which impairs the patients' quality of life and reinforces the stigma.

Fernandes and others (2007) in their study found out that the magnitude of stigma is different within segments of the local society, highlighting that socio-cultural factors such as gender, religion, and level of education may be important predictor of stigma. They also found out that the areas most affected by epilepsy stigma were work and social relationships. Studies in Europe and North America suggest that the stigma of epilepsy is one of the most important negative influences on the quality of life of the people with epilepsy. Baker, 2002, Fisher, et al., 2000; Baker, et al., 1997 in an European study found that people felt that epilepsy and its treatment affected their daily lives and their perceived health status. This study highlighted the impact of epilepsy on relationships, social life, employment, and plans for the future. Furthermore, more than 50% of people with epilepsy reported feelings of stigma. In a British study (Jacoby, et al., 2004) suggested that, in general, people who know someone with epilepsy more often believe that people with epilepsy have more personality difficulties than others.

In a survey study in Estonia (Herodes, et al., 2001) found that epilepsy influenced employment opportunities, as well as social functioning, physical and emotional aspects, general health, and vitality. In another study in China (Kleinman, et al., 1995) pointed out that epilepsy has consequences on family, marriage, financial, moral and social aspects of the patient's life. The social course of epilepsy depends on economic and social factors, and, for this reason, the stigma can be heterogeneous and changeable.

Unemployment and underemployment exist world-wide, but more so with people with epilepsy. The misunderstanding and stigma mentioned previously are usually to blame for this. For instance, a survey in China showed that 30% of respondents believe that people with epilepsy should not be employed. Data from German, Italy and United States of America indicate that people with epilepsy of working age, 40% - 60% are employed (although these jobs are below their potential), 15% - 20% are unemployed and about 20% retire early. In a recent research survey, nearly a quarter of Nepaless people with epilepsy took to the view that they were unable to work. As in many countries, these people with epilepsy had been culturally conditioned to underrate themselves.

From all indications, self-esteem of the epileptic patients could be badly affected because of their condition. The researcher perceived that the rejection of epileptic patients and the psychosocial problems experienced by them could bring about low self-esteem. Self-esteem, a part of self-concept is a personal judgement about self – worth, value and competence in other words, how a person feels about self. To increase self-esteem of individuals, with low self-esteem, researchers have found that four main strategies help to improve self-esteem. For example (i) identifying the cause of low self-esteem (ii) experiencing emotional support (iii) achieving and (iv)coping (Bednar, Wells & Peterson, 1995; Harter, 1998). Some psychologists asserts that the most effective ways to improve self-esteem is to improve the person's achievement, coping skills and counselling to improve their general well-being.

A chronic disease such as epilepsy can be an important stress factor, and inability to deal with the condition can bring psychological difficulties and emotional discomfort. These difficulties and emotional discomfort include, recurrent seizures, restrictions on normal activities such as driving, swimming, working with machine in industries, resulting to higher incidence of unemployment. Additional stressors associated with the illness include the psychological consequences of coping with repeated episodes of loss of consciousness often associated with embarrassment and loss of personal dignity. The uncertainty of never knowing when or where the seizure will occur, lowers the patient's self-esteem, lead to consequent breakdown of mental function. The presence of these inherent psychosocial problems makes epileptic patients liable to the development of psychiatric distress (Olley, 1997). Adult epileptic patients are particularly at risk as they will be unable to provide for the family as a result of the illness.

Individuals with epilepsy suffer discrimination, a higher incidence of unemployment difficulties, social exclusion, lower marital rates and are predisposed to cognitive impairment due to cerebral damage and/or antiepileptic medication, Santrock (2003). Other psychosocial problems include low self-esteem, stigma, negative self-concept, distorted interpersonal adjustment, alienation from both family and the society and psychiatric illness which include depression, anxiety and psychosis.

Epilepsy commonly affects young people in the most productive years of their lives, often leading to avoidable unemployment. The unemployed epileptic patients tend to become depressed, morose, apathetic, aggressive and demoralized, which may precipitate fits. Many adolescents with epilepsy face an uncertain and possible hostile environment because caregivers thought that epilepsy was contagious or a form of mental illness and these adolescents might be socially isolated as a result of peer ignorance. Both men and women face several social difficulties due to public image of persons with seizure. Fear, horror, superstition, prejudice and erroneous beliefs hold true even today to the epileptics. This is more so in the case of a girl/woman, who may not be accepted as a wife even to the enlightened educated persons including doctors, psychologist and other highly placed men in the society. Male epileptic patients may not be accepted by any young woman for marriage because of epileptic disorder the man is experiencing. This has brought untold hardship to the epileptic patients in our society.

RECOMMENDATIONS

Psycho-education is recommended for the treatment of epileptic patients especially the chronic ones who could not respond to antiepileptic drugs. There should be awareness to the caregivers about epileptic disorder and campaign against people discriminating against those with epilepsy since it is like any other disease people suffer from in the society (for example hypertension, diabetes, asthma etcetera and are not transferred to others).

The treatment strategies reviewed in this study are recommended for use by psychologies and medical professional for proper assessment, diagnosis, planning, implementation and evaluation. These groups include epileptics with poorly controlled seizures, high perceived stigma, poor emotional, vocational, interpersonal, marital and poor adjustments to seizure respectively. This in line with Olley (1997) findings, that the epileptic patients have poor controlled seizures high perceived stigma, poor emotional vocational, interpersonal, marital and poor adjustment to seizures. The management of epileptic patients should consist of the physicians, neurologist, psychiatrist, clinical psychologist, social workers, counselling psychologists, nurses and alternative medicine specialists.

Social support is very important in the lives of epileptic patients to minimize the stressors imposed on them by this chronic disease (epilepsy). The single and unemployed epileptics need support from family members, philanthropist and government of this country. Sheltered workshops should be built and these patients employed to fern for themselves and where they will be properly managed. Vocational training is suggested for young epileptic patients where they will be given special training for betterment of their lives in adulthood/old age.

This study is recommended for policy makers in health industry to serve as an input on mental health issues relating to improvement of the lives of epileptics, to embark on campaign against discriminating people with epileptic disorders (stigma) and accept them as other citizens.

REFERENCES

Ablon, J. 2002 The nature of stigma and medical conditions. *Epilepsy Behaviour 2002:* 3 6, suppl. 2: 2-9.

Ackner, B. 2005. Handbook for Psychiatric Nurses. 14th Edition, London. Tindall and Cassel.

Alloy, L. B; Jacobson, N. S and Acocella, J 1999. *Abnormal psychology current perspectives* 8th Ed. McGraw-Hill. Boston.

Awaretefe A. Longe A. C and Awaretefe M. 1985a. Epilepsy and psychosis, A comparison of Social attitudes, international league against Epilepsy. *Epilepsia*, 26(1); 1-9. Raven press, New-York.

Barraclough, B Suicide and Epilepsy. In Reynolds, E. H, Trimble, MR – eds Epilepsy and Psychiatry. Edinburgh: *Churchill Livingstone, 1982: 72-85.*

Barry, K. 1982. The health education needs of the adult with epilepsy. *Rehabilitation nursing. 7: 30-33.*

Berman, A; Snyder, S. J. Kozier, B, and Erb, G. 2008. *Kozier and Erb's Fundamentals of Nursing concepts, process and practice*, 8th Edition. Upper Saddle River. New Jersey.

Bhatia 2010a, *Essentials of Psychiatry* 6th Edition, C135 Publishers and Distributors Pv, Ltd. New Delhi.

Blume W, Luders H, Mizrahi E, Tassinaric, Van Emde Boas w, Engel J 2001. "Glossary of descriptive terminology for ictal semiology: report of the ILAE task force on classification and terminology" *Epilepsia 42 (9): 1212-8, do: 10, 1046/j. 1528 – 1157. 2001. 2200. X PMID 11580774.*

Cross, C. 2004. Seizures. *Regaining control* RN, 67 (12), 44-50.

Dada, T. O. 1970. Epilepsy in Lagos, *Nigeria African journal of medical sciences* 1:76-84.

Devinsky, O. 2008 Easing the seizures and stigma of epilepsy NY Times. Com.

Fernandes P. T, Salgdo PC, Noronha ALA, De Boer HM, Prilopko L, Sander JW & L. M. L. 2007 Epilepsy stigma perception in an urban area of a limited resource country *Epilepsy & Behaviour*11, 25 – 32.

Fisher R, Van ende Boas, Blum W, Genton P. Leep, Engel J 2005. "Epileptic seizures and epilepsy: definitions proposes by the international League Against Epilepsy (ILAE) and the International Bureau for Epilepsy (IBE)" *Epilepsia* 46 (4): 470-2 doi: 11 11/j. 0013 – 9580. 2005, 66104.x. PMID 15816939.

Frucht, M. M. Quigg M. Schwaner C. Fountain N. B 2000 "Distribution of seizure precipitants among epilepsy syndromes. *Epilepsia*41(12)1534- 1539.

Gelder M Harrison, P., cowen P 2006 Shorter Oxford Text book of psychiatry, fifth edition, New York. Oxford University press Inc.

Harter, S. 1998. The Development of Self-Representations. In W. Damon (ed.) *Handbook of Child Psychology* (5th ed., vol. 3). New York: Wiley. II.

Hausa, W. A, Kurland, L. T. 1975 "The epidemiology of epilepsy in Rochester, Minnesota, 1935 through 1967" *Epilepsia*16 (1): 1-66.doi;llll/j.1528-1157.1975.tb04721.x (http;//dx. dvoi.org/10.llll%2fj.1157.1975.tb0472.x). PMID 804401 (//www.ncbi.nlm.nih.gov/ pubmed/804401).

Herodes M. Oun A, Hidres, Kaasik AE 2001. Epilepsy in Estonia: a quality of life study. *Epilepsia* 42: 1061-73.

Hills, M. D. 2007. The Psychological and Social impact of epilepsy. *Neurology Asia*; 12 (Supplement 1): 10-12.

Hirtz, D. Thurman, D. J. Ginn-Hardy, K, Mohammed, M. Chaudhuri, A. R. Zalutsky, R. 2007. "How common are the 'commons' neurological disorders? Neurology 68 (5):326-37…. (//www.nci.nlm.nih.gov/pubmed/17261678).

Hosie, B 2007. Cognitive and Psychosocial problems in children with epilepsy A population-based approach. Institute of Clinical Medicine, Section for pediatrics and institute of Biological and medical psychology. University of Bergen, Norway. http://www.intercom. net/npo/eaes/facts.htm.

Jacoby, A, Snape D, Baker G. A. Epilepsy and social identity the stigma of a chronic neurological disorder. *Lancet Neural* 2005; 4: 171-8.

Kleinman A, Wang WZ, L: Sc, et al. 1995. The social course of epilepsy chronic illness as social experience in interior China. *Soc. Sci Med 1995*; 40: 1319-30.

Loeser, J. D. & Howe J. F. 1980. Differentiation and neuronal injury. *In epilepsy. A window to Brain Mechanisms*. pp 123-133. New York, Raven Press.

Lovely, M. P and Ozuma J. 1986. Status epilepitus. In Nikas D (Ed). *The critically ill neuro surgical patient,* pp 125-139. Edinburg, Churchill-Livingstone.

MacLeod, J. S & Austin, J. K. 2003. Stigma in the lives of adolescents with epilepsy: a review of the literature. *Epilepsy Behaviour* 4: 112-7.

Meldrum B. 1982. Pathology and pathophysiology: *In Laidlow J. Richens A.* (ed). A Textbook of *Epilespy*, pp 456-487. Edinburgh, Churchill. Livingstone.

Meldrum B., 1978. Physiological changes during prolonged seizures and epileptic brain damage. *Neuropediatric* 9(3) 203-212.

Mendel, G. 1986 VersucheuberFlanzenhybriden (Experiment in plant hybridization). *Vereines in Bruenn*, 4,3-47.

National Institute of Mental Health 2007. The 2007 National Survey of Mental Health and wellbeing. www.aihw.gov.au/mental-health.

National Institute of Neurological Disorders and Stroke, 2010).
Olley, B. O. 1997. Psychosocial determinant of interictal psychopathology and efficacy of psychoeducation in Nigeria epileptics. PhD Thesis.
Osuntokun, B. O. & Odeku, E. L. 1970. Some aspects of epilepsy in Nigerians. *Tropical Geographical Medicine*, 22: 3-19.
Osuntokun, B. O. 1971. Epilepsy in the developing countries: The Nigeria profile. *Epilespia*. 12: 107-111.
Osuntokun, B. O.; Adeuja, A. O. G. Nottidge V. A. Bademosi 1987. Prevalence of the Epilepsies in Nigeria Africans: A Community Based Study. *Epilepsia*. 28: 272-279.
Ozuma, J and Cammermeyer, m. 1983 Epilepsy, A course syllabus independent study. University of Washington, Seattle.
Ozuma, J. 1979. Psychosocial aspect of epilepsy. *Journal of Neurosurgery Nursing*. 11:242-246.
Ozuna, J. 1981. Compliance with therapeutic regimens: Issues, answers, and research questions. *J. Neurosurg Nurs* 13 (1) 1-6.
Ozuna, J. 1986. Compliance with therapeutic regimens: Issues, answers, and research questions. *J. Neurosurg Nurs* 13 (1) 1-6.
Ozuna, J. Commermeyer M: 1983. Epilepsy: A course syllabus for independent study: University of Washington Seattle.
Pond, D. 1981. Psychosomatic aspect of epilepsy. In Rose F. C. (ed). Research Progress in epilepsy. London: Atmon Books; 175-480.
Santrock, J. W. 2003. Psychology, 7th Edition., McGraw-Hill Companies Inc. Boston.
Scambler, G. & Hopkins, A. 1980. Social Class, epileptic activity, and disadvantage at work. *Journal of Epidemiology Community Health*. 34: 129-133.
Scambler, G; Hopkins, A. 1986 Being epileptic: Coming to terms with stigma. *Soc. Health Illness*: 8: 26-43.
Scambler G, Hopkins A., 1990 Generating a model of epileptic stigma the role of qualitative analysis. *Social Science Medical* 30 1187-94.
Shorvan, S. 1990. Epilepsy: A Lancet Review London: The Lancet.
Shorvan, S. 2000. Handbook of Epilepsy Treatment Blackwell Science Ltd Oxford.
Solomon, C. & Jackson – Jobe, P. 1992. Helping homeless people: unique challenge and solutions. Alexandria, V. A. American Association for Counselling and Development.
Solomon, C. Kutt, H., Plum F: 1983. Clinical management of seizures Philadelphia, WB.
Trethowan, J. 2002. Psychiatry. 10th Edition. Balliere Tindall & Cassel London.
Walsh, M. 2005. Watson's clinical nursing and related sciences. 6th edition. BaillereTindall. Edinburgh.
Watson J. E 2005. Caring science as sacred science. *Philadephia*: F. A. Davis.
Watson, J. E. & Royle, J. R. 2002. Watsons Medical-Surgical Nursing and Related *Physiology* 5th Edition. Bailliere – Tindall, London.
Wells, L. E and G. Marwell. 1976. Self-Esteem: Its Conceptualization and Measurement. Beverly Hills, Calif.: Sage.
World Health Organization 2012. Epilepsy: Fact sheet number 999. Retrieved Nov. 12, 2013, from http://www.int/mediacentre/factsheets/fs999/en/.
Wyler, A & Ward, A. A: 1980. *Epileptic neurosis*. In epilepsy, *A window to Brain mechanisms*, pp 51-68. New York, Raven Press.

In: Caregivers
Editor: Adrienne Lloyd

ISBN: 978-1-63483-909-9

Chapter 4

AN EXPLORATORY STUDY OF PARENTS' PERCEIVED NEEDS IN CARING FOR A CHILD WITH LEARNING DISABILITIES

Wai Tong Chien
School of Nursing, Faculty of Health and Social Sciences
The Hong Kong Polytechnic University, Hong Kong S.A.R., P.R. China

ABSTRACT

Caring for a child with learning difficulties can be both a rewarding and a difficult experience; however, little is known about parents' perceptions of caring for these children and their psychosocial well-being. This exploratory, qualitative study was conducted to explore these couples' perceived health needs in care-giving to a child with different learning difficulties (LD). A purposive sample of 22 couples who were caring for a child with LD at home were recruited from two regional child mental health centers in Hong Kong. Data were collected from individual couples with semi-structured interviews between April and June 20134. Each interview was audio-taped and lasted more than one hour. These interview data were transcribed to Chinese and analyzed by using content analysis. Four categories of parents' perceived health needs were identified, including needs for specific knowledge (and skills) about care provision, health issues of self and LD child, showing much demands for psychosocial support, and barriers to seeking helps and support. Specific health needs related to knowledge of the illness and its care, social support from spouse and health professionals, and reluctance to seek help from people were perceived as important by the parents. These results reveal important issues and challenges in providing illness- and culture-specific nursing care for these family carers. The findings can facilitate health professionals understand parental needs with regard to knowledge of the illness, psychosocial support, expectations to their child, and attitude and behavior towards help-seeking in LD caregiving. Health care providers should provide appropriate education for these families in terms of their psychosocial and culture-specific needs, in order to improve their health and well-being.

Keywords: family health, learning disabilities, parenting, qualitative exploratory study

BACKGROUND OF THE STUDY

Learning disabilities or difficulties (LD) in childhood refers to a group of mental disorders characterised by difficulties in learning some basic academic skills that are not consistent with the person's chronological age, educational opportunities or intellectual abilities (American Psychiatric Association, 2000). Children with this disorder may often manifest disturbing behaviours such as agitation and temper tantrums and these disturbances significantly interfere with their activities of daily living. Its onset is usually over the infancy or childhood stage and is attributed by information processing deficits of parts of central nervous system (Karande, Mehta, and & Kulkami, 2007). According to Lam (2005), there are mainly four sub-types of SLD, including dyslexia, language disorder, dyscalculia, and non-verbal learning (e.g., visual-spatial and motor coordination) disability.

In the United States, about 15% of the population have been suffered from different types of learning difficulties, most having a need for special education (Karande and Kulkarni, 2009). According to Smythe, Everatt and Salter (2003), the prevalence of dyslexia was about 6% and 10% of the population in Finland and Japan, respectively. Similar to the U.K., the prevalence rate of SLD in Hong Kong had increased 1.5 times in three years to 10% in 2007 (Chan et al., 2008), and even more rapidly risen in the next five years (2008-12). However, there is a lack of medium- and long-term measures worldwide, including legislation and policies relating to educational, medical and familial care for these children (Kendall et al., 2005).

Family environment and family members' attitude towards caregiving to children with LD are an integral part of the bio-psychosocial development of these children, particularly those with serious learning difficulties and special health needs. Smythe et al. (2003) suggested that educational or clinical treatment of LD without considering familial contexts and needs significantly reduces the chances of successful intervention outcomes. Since there have been few studies specifically related to parenting and parents' adaptations to their caregiving and daily functioning, there is a lack of understanding about parents' health and educational needs in taking care of a child with LD, particularly in Asian and Chinese populations.

IMPACTS ON PARENTS IN TAKING CARING OF A CHILD WITH LEARNING DISABILITIES

Research has consistently indicated that family members in particular those parents who are caring for a child with intellectual and learning disabilities often experience higher levels of distress than those providing care for a normally developing child (Crnic, Gaze, and& Hoffman, 2005). According to Rayner and Moore (2007), both parents experienced similar levels of stress and poor social life in taking care of a difficult child because of the higher demands for caregiving, academic achievements, and inadequate psychosocial support secured from other family members and healthcare workers.

Recent studies on stress and difficulties facing by parents in caring for a child with LD or intellectual disabilities mainly focused on examining its related or predictive factors such as their socio-demographic and illness characteristics and socio-cultural environment. Keller and

Honig (2004) investigated the correlated factors of distress among 32 families with school-aged disabled children and found that these children's demands and neediness for care and problematic behaviors are strongly associated to their distress in caregiving. The considerable demands of managing these children's academic and life skills, sudden mood changes and challenging behaviors could further increase parents' caregiving stress (Phetrasuwan and & Miles, 2009). Fathers were found to become more stressed when they experienced negative attitudes and low social acceptance of their disabled children (Kenny and & McGillway, 2007).

While parenting can be rewarding and fulfilling, some evidence has suggested that parents experienced a wide range of negative physical, psychological and social effects in caring for a child with different disabilities (Crnic et al., 2005; Rayner and & Moore, 2007). Psychological impacts mainly include worry, anxiety and depression (Phetrasuwan and Miles, 2009), reduced self-esteem (Hill & Rose, 2009), and emotional pain, frustration and feelings of shame and guilt (Saloviita, Italinna & Leinonen, 2003). Heiman's (2002) interviewed 32 parents of children with LD in Israel indicated that they felt a low level of autonomy and self-efficacy in child care, and were dissatisfied with their parenting skills. The effects of caregiving on parents' physical health, such as gastrointestinal disturbance and weight reduction, are relatively less severe than its social effects, such as reduced social activities and poor interpersonal relationships (Crnic et al., 2005).

Parents' Health Needs in Caregiving to a Child with LD

The earliest study conducted by Waggoner and Wilgosh (1990) who explored eight parents' concerns about caring for their child with learning disability at home. The parents indicated getting emotionally and physically drained due to their time demanding involvements in their child's education, and facing negative experiences with the school personnel who were perceived to be uncooperative and misunderstanding with their child's problems. A literature review by Griffiths, Bennet, and Smith (2008) on 180 research studies on LD recommended that most of studies relevant to parents' caregiving to their ill children were small-scale qualitative research, cross-sectional descriptive surveys or service evaluation, which do not in themselves constitute a sufficient body of research evidence to inform or support the design of effective interventions for these people and their families. Although 55 studies focused on the family carers of people with LD, particularly parents and siblings, they had small sample sizes of 10-15 parents and used focus groups to explore recent experiences and needs for service utilization. A few quantitative, descriptive studies also raised the issue of cultural beliefs in taking care of these children with LD and recommended further investigation of this important subject in future research (Azar & Badr, 2006; Little & Clark, 2006). To address the health needs and demands of parents and other family caregivers in LD, more exploratory research should be conducted for a better and in-depth understanding of these parents' or carers' health concerns and educational needs with regard to caregiving.

Compared with research on children with various physical and intellectual disabilities, there are few studies on parents' perceived health concerns and educational needs in caring for a child with LD. Only a few studies have been found to examine parents' coping with stress in relation to care-giving. An U.S. survey conducted by Little (2002) on coping strategies among parents of children with non-verbal learning disorders indicated that mothers were more likely than fathers to seek help from health professionals, improve their coping skills or sharing with relatives. In addition, Chang and Hsu's (2007) exploratory study on 117 Taiwanese families found that care-giving to children with learning disorders is a complex process of familial adjustment. Interestingly, support from their religion was indicated as an important spiritual support among these Chinese families, thus highlighting the potential significance of socio-cultural factors influencing family coping with care-giving. In view of limited studies found, there is a lack of understanding about parents' health needs in caring for a child with LD. Keller and Honig (2004) suggested that relatively more time and energy are spent on parenting children with LD than on those without any behavioral or learning problems. In addition, the parents' difficulties in accepting the diagnosis of the illness and their child's learning and social difficulties were also considered a major problem.

Although more than half of the recent research on LD has focused on family health, few studies have been found that examine parents' help-seeking behaviors and coping with regard to caregiving. According to the cognitive appraisal of stress and ways of coping suggested by the Cognitive Appraisal Model (Lazarus, 1991), these families' perception of stress in caregiving and its related coping behaviors are important in understanding the health and well-being of the family caregivers, as well as family-centered care of these children with LD (Griffiths et al., 2009). A U.S. survey conducted by Little (2002) on coping strategies among parents of children with nonverbal learning disorders indicated that mothers were more likely than fathers to seek help from health professionals or share with relatives. In addition, Chang and Hsu's (2007) exploratory study of 117 Taiwanese families found that caregiving for children with learning disorders was a complex process of familial adjustment. The support from their religion or traditional Chinese beliefs such as Confucianism and Taoism were found to provide important spiritual support to these Chinese families, highlighting the significance of socio-cultural factors on family coping with caregiving. However, the effects of culture and subtypes of SLD are unclear, with limited research evidence of their effects on parenting and family health, especially in Asian populations (Ho, Chien & Wang, 2011; Lam, 2005). Therefore, this study was to explore Chinese parents' perception and understanding about LD and its care, as well as their perceived health needs and hindrances encountered in their child care. The findings are useful to provide better understanding about these parents' caregiving needs and design effective intervention for meeting these demands and needs.

METHODS

Study Design

A descriptive qualitative study approach was used in exploring Chinese parents' perceived health needs and concerns in caring for a child with LD in Hong Kong. This approach enables the natural yielding of useful insights and an in-depth understanding of a social phenomenon (Denzin & Lincoln, 2005), such as parents' perceptions of their caregiving in this study.

Participants and Study Setting

In this study, we recruited a purposive sample of 22 pairs of Chinese parents who were caring for a child diagnosed with LD from two regional child mental health centers in the largest geographical region of Hong Kong. These centers served >2,000 children with different developmental disorders (i.e., 20% of the total population of LD in 2010, as reported by The Hong Kong Association of [Specific] Learning Disabilities, 2010), and their families. Its family services included mainly comprehensive health assessment, medical treatment, referrals to medical, mental health and social services, and psychosocial interventions such as social skills training.

The purposive sampling used was the best means of selection and recruitment of the most appropriate informants with a maximum variation of characteristics specific and important to elicit the most information about the topic, thus best answering the research questions (Munhall, 2007). For instance, parents with different ages, education levels and/or duration of care-giving were recruited to explore a diverse variety of perceived health needs from their common and unique caring experiences at different illness stages.

As suggested by Bowen (2008) and Morse (2000), 15 to 20 participants would allow for rich and in-depth data collection via semi-structured interviews and provide the possibility for achieving data saturation, which is the point in data collection and analysis where no new ideas arise. With the concurrent data collection and data analysis approach, the achievement of data saturation was subsequently checked and reached during content analysis when 16 21 couples had been interviewed (hence, interviews with 22 couples were finally conducted).

The inclusion criteria for the parents in the study were:

i) aged 18 or above and able to speak Cantonese or Mandarin;
ii) Hong Kong Chinese residents;
iii) biological mothers and fathers who were living with and caring for a child with LD; and
iv) primary carers who played the main role in looking after the child;

Parents were excluded from this study if they had a known history of psychiatric, cognitive or acute medical illness, a child with LD under court order, or if they had known about their child's illness or undertaken the care-giving role for <1 month.

Data Collection

The participants were recruited from April through June 2014. The study was approved by the Human Subjects Research Ethics Committee of The Hong Kong Polytechnic University and the study centre. The researchers checked the family's and child's particulars in the computerised clinical records of the two centres against the study criteria, and formed a list of eligible participants. The confidentiality of the data was assured with no discussion about the interview content or data with any center staff and informing each of the right to withdraw from the study at anytime without any negative consequence on their care to be received. The author then selected two pairs of parents from the list with diverse characteristics in terms of their education level and duration of caregiving. The selected parents were contacted via phone, given a full explanation of the study and invited by one researcher to participate in the study. After their written consent had been obtained, they were interviewed at a time and venue convenient to them. After content analysis of these three interviews, the subsequent 19 pairs of parents were selected from the same parent list according to the preliminary categories that emerged, and further information needed to clarify the important issues was identified.

Table 1. Interview Guide for Parents of Children with Learning Difficulties

Questions	Examples of probes
1. In caring for your child with LD, please describe:	
• Your everyday caregiving to the child	- Personal hygiene and care - School and academic work - Leisure and activities - Other learning activities
• What you know about LD	- Diagnosis, etiology treatment, and prognosis - Main characteristics of SLD and learning problems
• What you think and feel about your caregiving	- Your feeling when learned the diagnosis - Thinking about the caregiving required - Your recent conditions and thoughts
2. What you expect to know about your caregiving	- Caring for the illness - Daily personal care - Academic performance - Family affairs and activities
3. Any information you received from the doctor, nurse, other health professionals, or teachers?	- Doctor's advice and treatment prescribed - Nursing care, e.g., family care and ADL - Teachers' advices on schooling - Any counselling and community support services
4. What are your concerns and comments on caregiving?	- Physical health and illness - Psychological and emotional - Family and social support - Personal and community resources
5. Please describe one or two recent experiences of child care that have made the deepest impression.	
- Any challenges or difficulties you encountered in care-giving - Ways for dealing with difficulties or challenges. Any examples?	- Health and well-being - Employment - Academic work - Recreation and activities - Family relationships
6. Do you think you have received adequate information and support for caregiving? What additional information/support needed?	

Semi-structured interviews were used to collect data from individual couples using an interview guide designed by the researchers. This interview method can encourage participants to discuss their own needs, concerns and difficulties encountered, thus facilitating an understanding of their perceived health needs in a specific context (Burns and & Grove, 2010). During each couple interview, both mother and father were encouraged to give their opinions on each question. When one was found dominant in discussion, the other who was passive and less responsive would be asked to answer the interview question first. The interview guide (Table 1) was designed on the basis of recent literature and the researchers' clinical expertise in the family care of children with LD (Ho et al., 2011). To assess the clarity, appropriateness and adequacy of the questions used, the guide was reviewed by an expert panel, including one child psychiatrist, two advanced practice psychiatric nurses, one psychiatric nurse educator, and two parents with relevant care-giving experiences. The panel commented that the questions were clear and adequate for exploration of the parents' health needs. All the interviews were conducted in Cantonese by the author, lasting 45-60 minutes and audio-taped with the parents' permission.

Data Analysis Procedure

The author and an experienced qualitative researcher independently undertook the transcription and translation (from Cantonese/Mandarin to English) of the first two interviews. The quality of translation was then checked by the second (bilingual) author. A high level of agreement between two translators on the transcripts was reported and only a few minor changes such as the terminologies to describe feelings were made. After all transcripts had been checked, content analysis was adopted to analyze the interview data (Graneheim & Lundman, 2004). All the data obtained were first read sentence by sentence by the author in order to determine their key concepts and meaning. The data were then analyzed by meaning units, which could be words, phrases or sentences. Meaningful entities were identified related to parents' perceptions, feelings and any concerns about caregiving, psychosocial well-being, and what information and services and resources they needed for caregiving. Each interview was segmented by these units, which were labelled by codes by the first author and one research assistant independently. To enhance objectivity and reduce threats to the trustworthiness of category development, consensuses on the meaningful units and codes were made between both investigators before performing any categorization. This was found to achieve 95% coding agreement, indicating very satisfactory consensus on the codes produced (Gilstrap, 2004). After repeated comparisons between codes in one interview and between interviews, categories and sub-categories were identified. These categories that emerged were discussed and also agreed, with a few minor amendments made on the wordings of the subcategories. Category/subcategory matching, condensation and finalizing were then performed, accommodating diverse experiences, comments and concerns from each of the 22 couples. Finally, the first author compared and contrasted the finalised finalized categories and subcategories between genders.

Results

Characteristics of Participants

We interviewed 21 couples, among whom one couple was unable to attend the interview due to time constraints. Their ages ranged from 28 to 45, with a mean of 31.5 years (SD = 6.0). 17 Seventeen mothers and 16 fathers (78.6%) had secondary school education or above, and 12 couples (57%) had religion or traditional (ancestor) worshipping behaviors. Eleven couples (57%) had two or more children, and mean duration of caregiving was 20.8 months (SD = 12.3), ranging from 5-34 months. Among the 21 mothers, six were in full-time employment and seven were part-time clerical workers. Sixteen fathers had full-time employment (in service and manual skill sectors), and the remaining five worked in part-time mode.

All of the children with LD were in the first to sixth years of primary school and more than half were boys (n = 14, 67%). Their median age was 6.3 years, ranging from 6-14. The duration of their illness ranged from 5-46 months, with a mean of 18.53 months (SD = 14.81). Most of them (n = 16, 76%) were diagnosed with two types of LD such as dyslexia, developmental coordination disorder and/or perceptual disorder and three (14%) were with multiple types.

Major Categories/Subcategories of Parents' Caregiving Needs

The four major categories and its sub-categories are identified and described at below. One category, obstacles that hindered help-seeking, was identified particularly by a few mothers, revealing specific cultural issues.

Needs for Specific Information about Care Provision

Most of the parents described LD to be the "difficulties or problematic behaviors in learning daily living skills, academic ability and self-care" as manifested by their children with the intellectual or learning disorder(s). However, none of them could explain the nature and underlying causes of LD. They informed us that the main sources of information about the illness were received from other parents, their family members and relatives, and internet and online resources. Only two young couples had acquired important information of the illness from psychiatrists and other mental health workers. Most of the couples indicated *a high level of immediate need for understanding the illness and its treatment/care*. For example, one young father said,

> "I thought LD was the child kept jumping, shouting and non-stop moving from time to time, was unable to interact verbally in a clear and systematic manner with other people... and very poor academic performance. After we consulted a psychiatrist, I realize my daughter had some learning difficulties due to developmental or neurological problems. I had never thought about the causes of this illness and its treatment needed..." (Parent 05, paragraph 8, lines 3-7)

With their limited knowledge of LD, most of them expressed *a need for better understanding and learning the skills in assisting their child's academic and living skills.* While most children showing multiple types of LD and thus difficulties in performing diverse self-care and interpersonal functions, academic skills such as calculation and reading and writing sentences, and expressing feelings and emotions appropriately. Many of them did recognized that these child characteristics or abilities were very different between children with LD even at similar ages but they did not know "how to assist and help these (my) children." Most mothers who were much committed and full-time involved in caring for their children at home reflected that they spent very long periods (i.e., 5-6 hours) everyday to teach or assist their children to complete all homework and revisions. They often lost their tempers when their children were not concentrated and did not listen to them, and also "when the child was scored very low in tests or assessments."

Despite these parents often felt frustrated and disappointed, most of them expressed *a strong desire to learn and adapt effective parenting*; however, they did not know how to achieve this. For example, one father mentioned that "…I have been spending all my time teaching my son after work but in vain. I would like to have somebody telling me how to teach… or at least listen to others for the ways to improve the child's attention and study ability." (Parent 07, paragraph 11, m lines 7-8).

Health Issues of Self and the LD Child

Most parents expressed a wide variety of health issues in relation to their caregiving. They were not only concerned about *physical health of themselves and their children but also their psychosocial conditions.* It seemed that these health issues are inter-related complex condition, reflecting a need for holistic view and support for these families. Although there were a few positive gains mentioned by these parents, those negative caregiving experiences such as incidents of failure in modifying their child's behaviors and hopelessness about the prognosis of LD in their children. For those with full-time employment, their main physical health issues were exhaustion, fatigue, poor quality of sleep, and general aches and discomfort. Many parents also indicated that they were very anxious and stressful, considering the life situations in negative manners, and lack of interest and motivation in social and recreational activities. Younger parents viewed these concerns to be in the highest priorities, in which family relationships, social interaction and work, as well as sexual behavior, were also affected. A few younger parents expressed much concerns with their social activities and relationships such as social life restrictions, increased conflicts with people and reduced social networks, mainly due to very much time and energy and thus high demands for caregiving; they often felt self-blame for responsibility to the illness and inadequacy of caregiving. One young woman said,

> "I have already exert most time and energy in caring for my daughter with dyslexia and disturbing behaviors and thus put aside other recreational and family activities performed prior to caregiving. This appears to disrupt all of my social life but I understand I need to take care of my beloved child. I can't leave my spouse or family members to do this alone." (Parent 11, paragraph 35).

A few main concerns with their child were expressed by these parents. Majority of them showed *disappointment and frustration about the academic performance of their children* and highlighted that many school teachers could not understand their children (or the illness) and special care for learning difficulties. School teachers were found to disparage their children's performance in class and feel unsatisfied with "discouraging remarks" such as poor concentration, unmotivated and lazy. Without any special consideration taken for their children, school teachers were described to be "often not understand their children's specific learning and caring needs," and thus any disturbed moods or behavior of their children was blamed and punished. They emphasized that this misunderstanding and mistreat would much affect their children's learning and psychosocial development.

Even though the children and parents worked very hard together, these children's academic performance was unsatisfactory or fluctuating. These parents believed that academic performance was very important to contribute and predict their children's future success and prospects. Most parents were worried about "whether my child can live and work independently or even earn his living in future." Many of them felt ambivalent about choosing a secondary school (with ordinary/special education curriculum) for their children. What one mother of a son, aged 10, with specific learning disability can illustrate this below:

> "My son is now studying in primary five and it is time to think about an appropriate secondary school for him... Many friends told me that most ordinary secondary schools would not accept a child with LD, and that many teachers was not good at teaching children with special education needs... I think it is very difficult to find a suitable school for him. His academic performance is not so good, I feel really disappointed and concerned about his future... after we (parents) both are dead." (Parent 13, paragraph 61).

Showing Much Demands for Psychological and Social Support

Most of the parents expressed *limited family services available or accessible* to support their caregiving. Many young couples indicated that they received limited support and advices from school or community services, and no respite care available to relieve their burnouts. They questioned about where and who could be approached for health education and promotion in LD care. One father with an a aged 6 years6-year-old dyslexia daughter reported,

> "I don't' know whether there are community supportive services or education programs are available for us parents... I have sought help from school, medical social workers and nursing staff but very little information received from them . . . I wonder there might be some health professionals able to give us advice or support... since I have not yet met any." (Parent 10, paragraph 71)

Most of these parents indicated that they obtained *inadequate psychosocial support in caregiving*. They valued much on any psychological support received, especially empathetic listening, discussion and reassurance; one of the cited examples was that a mutual support group for family caregivers of children with various types of LD was established to share and learn from each other about their similar needs and demands and some effective ways for caregiving. They voiced out that this group program was one of very few similar supportive one that they could involve; they mostly perceived that many parents and their family members were not willing to discuss about their children with LD and its related problems and care in need. It is important and interesting to note that most parents valued greatly the importance of spousal support but most were not so supportive or helpful in child care. For example, one younger mothers said,

> "I wish his (the son) father could have participated more in caring for him with much learning difficulties. For example, sharing some household chores and helping oru son to finish his homework... but he seems unhelpful so far. My husband often said he was so busy to work out his office work.... so he slept early. His comforting words and encouragement might also help me... to do the caregiving task with greater strengths and pleasure." (Parent 30, paragraph 18)

Barriers to Seeking Help and Support

Majority of them indicated that they were *reluctant to seek help from people* who were unfamiliar ones or not their close relatives or friends. It was due to their feeling of embarrassment and shameful or even guilty; they considered such help-seeking would make them and their family '*lose face*' (less respectable or feeling ashamed). One middle-aged mother stated,

> "My neighbors would not know our family affairs and problems and they might not be able to understand my daughter's LD. They might think that my daughter was strange, challenging and ridiculous . . . We would feel embarrassed and ashamed to ask them to help. I don't want my neighbors or friends to look upon us or treat us to be insane" (Parents 17, paragraph 45)

All parents felt *reluctant to talk about their child's illness and family needs*. They believed that they were responsible for family caregiving and comforting, thus reiterating a lot about seldom discussing about their children and the LD with friends, school staff and other parents of the same school. They were much concerned with "losing respect and social standing from their social groups." In addition, they also believed that these 'outsiders' could not understand their problems or difficulties and thus perceive them as "trouble-making" or "nonsense." Therefore even they felt very stressful, they were unwilling to and afraid of neither "asking questions about child care" nor "seeking advices on their life difficulties and management" of their children's challenging behaviors.

DISCUSSION

There are only very few research like this study to examine parents' information and perceived health needs in taking care of a child with learning disabilities. The findings in this exploratory study indicate that a few domains of educational needs were similar to those of family caregivers of children with developmental disorders, including psychologically highly stressful and hardship in the process of caregiving, lack of knowledge of the illness and preparation for skills or demands for caregiving, unrealistic expectations to the child with abnormal behaviors and different pathways of development, and inadequate family support resources (Buschgens et al., 2008; Chien et al., 2006; Ho et al., 2011). The findings also reveal a few major concerns of these parents such as inadequate social and spousal support and culture-specific high expectations of academic performance and future career in Hong

Kong, and much reluctance to seek help or ask questions from others in relation to 'face saving' or keeping the respect and dignity. These factors can play important roles in understanding the chronic illness and its long-term home care, as well as familial responses to caregiving and other life situations.

It appears that these parents would prefer to use problem-focused coping with their caregiving stress. According to Lazarus and Folkman (1984), this approach to coping means to face with the problem (stressor) and solve it directly by identifying the problem, evaluating alternatives, implementing strategies, and then seeking support and information. LD is a life-long challenging and deficit-type of problem for both children and their families. In addition to accept the medical diagnosis and thinking positively, the parents would have to face and resolve, or sometimes reduce or live with, the related life difficulties. Seeking relevant information and caregiving skills is an appropriate and effective way, as suggested by some of the parents in this study, to be the first step to problem-focused coping with their caring role.

Educational Needs for Family Caregiving

The parents indicated that they were not well-equipped with the knowledge and skills in caring for their children with LD and its health-related concerns, thus indicating uncertain about the ways for better caring for their children, and their well-being. Because of their limited knowledge of LD, they have not yet fully recognised the cognitive, emotional and behavioral problems manifested by their children at home and/or school, and could not work out the plan to get the children back to normal development. Perhaps, they might think their children had more deficits in bio-psychosocial development than other children with similar ages but they did not know the causative factors and prognosis of LD, thus resulting in unrealistic expectations of academic achievements towards their children. These parents who are unable to recognise the features and course of the illness are found to delay in assessment and treatment for their children with LD (Hill & Rose, 2009; Karande & Kulkarni, 2009).

Surprisingly, the parents indicated that they could not obtain appropriate and relevant information or support from health professionals, teachers and/or other parents to address their educational and psychosocial needs. Chien and Lee (2013) suggest that family caregivers of a child with developmental and/or learning problems are often ill-prepared for caregiving with limited knowledge and skills offered by health professionals and many questions about caregiving are unanswered such as the child's illness condition and behaviors, prognosis, the care required at home, and issues for studying at school and home settings. During the process of caregiving starting from knowing the clinical diagnosis of LD, the parents should undoubtedly need much information about the illness and its immediate and continuous medical treatment and most importantly, psychosocial care and behavioural management at home to deal with both daily personal, academic (or school) and family situations and activities. They should also need continuous practical assistance, psychosocial support and encouragement, and regular discussion or counselling about effective means or options for caregiving to their children with LD in long-term. Wide varieties of health-related issues and concerns in their caregiving and own psychosocial health reflect that there may be a need for more focused and specific health assessment and education to meet these families' bio-psychological needs.

The findings also revealed that these parents' coping with and use of family support resources available for caregiving to their children with LD were not addressed by mental healthcare system or any of the mental health professionals. The National Institute for Health and Clinical Excellence (NICE, 2008) suggested in the clinical guideline for management of learning disorders that person-centered care should be provided for these family or informal carers. In addition to the special care of children with LD, any treatment/intervention for the children with LD should take into account their family caregivers' needs and interests, from the perspective of these needy people. Effective and frequent communication between mental health professionals and these parents should be ensured and involvement of carers in any child care should be essential and thus reinforced in order to tailor evidenced-based psychosocial care and support to satisfy the holistic needs of these families.

Important Issues in Parenting a Child with LD Learning Disabilities (LD)

Contextually in Asian societies, Chinese parents of children with LD experienced wider varieties of difficult or stereotyped life situations, which may not be experienced by their Western counterparts. As suggested by early Western studies, physical and emotional disturbances are often reported by these parents due to demands for time and effort in caregiving and enhancing the academic performance of their children. With much emphasis and higher expectations towards academic performance and its impacts on future career, the parents in this study felt very disappointed, emotionally frustrated and sometimes giving up at times when they had experienced failures repeatedly in modifying those problematic behaviors of their children in daily activities, homework and revision, and school life. Gannon and McGilloway (2009) suggested that psychosomatic disturbances and agitation are more commonly experienced by carers or parents of a child with LD than those caring for a 'normal' child. Stigmatization to the children with LD and their families such as doing evil and disgraceful deeds in ancestors and current family members or parents can be easily found in Chinese communities to put the blame on the parents, or even the child, in causing the illness.

Particularly for those with full employment, taking care of a child with LD can much affect the carers' social lives such as regular family activities and hobbies and interpersonal relationships, thus reducing their quality of life in longer term (Keller and & Honig, 2004). A harmonious family relationship, which is crucial in mediating parental stress and facilitating child care, would be reduced or deterred if the carers could not have sufficient support and effective coping. In order to promote the quality of caregiving, these family caregivers' psychosocial health and well-being should be satisfied, in which mental health professionals should play an important role in needs assessment, problem diagnosis and intervention planning and evaluation at the earliest possible to meet these carers' health needs in LD care (Antshel & Joseph, 2006).

Moreover, social support in particular from intimate family members is considered an important mediating factors influencing caregiving burden and facilitating parents' coping with stress in caring for their children with developmental and learning disorders (Antshel & Joseph, 2006). The higher the level of perceived social support from family or spouse, the more the parents' satisfaction with their caregiving experiences and thus the lower their distress would be. In addition, psychological, emotional, and instrumental support or practical assistance with family chores and caring role are significant factors in reducing these carers' tensions and anxiety. Therefore, mental health professionals should provide appropriate education and instrumental support for these parents, concerning their skills in caregiving and mutual support between carers with similar situations in the community.

It is important but surprised to note that health professionals and school teachers are not equipped properly or adequately with both knowledge and skills in family care in LD. The parents were not educated and trained by mental health professionals in preparing them for LD caregiving. Similar to the findings in some Asian countries (e.g., Chan, 2008; Keller & Honig, 2004), most school staff such as teachers and nurses do not know how to educate students with LD appropriately. To enhance professional support for these parents, specialized LD care team should be set up to formulate appropriate training programs for these professional care providers who have direct contact with and care for these families to provide specific mental health assessment, education and support to the families of a child with LD.

Cultural Issues in LD Caregiving

A few cultural issues were identified in relation to parents' perceived difficulties in caregiving that might hinder their help-seeking or caregiving tasks. First, the Chinese parents indicated a much lower understanding of LD and less accessibility to family support services, when compared with those parents in developed Western countries. Teacher and parent training in special education and a school nurse with specialised skills in LD care are commonly found in schools in most developed countries, but rarely found in Hong Kong (Ngan Keung, 2008). Few organisations in Hong Kong are working for and implementing family-centered care for children with LD, even though LD is considered as a disabling problem in the community (Chien & Lee, 2013). Hence, the parents might find it really difficult to meet the developmental and learning needs of their children with LD.

Second, Chinese societies emphasises high academic achievement and career expectations and this study does reveals such kinds of social or cultural issues on both the children and their parents. High social demands and expectations to the children, in spite that they have learning disabilities, can result in high tensions or burden among the parents and transferred to the children with LD. Consequently, these high expectations would become emotional turmoil among the carers, turning out to be frequent disappointments, anger and frustration when their child fails to follow their teaching or get the satisfactory grade in study. Assessing the societal and familial expectations of children with LD and their impacts on parenting is essential to the health professionals to provide appropriate health promotion and education for these carers.

Third, traditional Chinese culture is important and influential in Chinese parents to follow the Confucian principles of courageously persevering and 'keeping the problems inside family' in the face of difficulty, rather than potentially disrupting stable relations with others, especially the unfamiliar ones or outsiders (Chang & Hsu, 2007). The majority of parents in this study could hide up or suppress their ideas potentially attributing to 'losing face' (i.e., losing the honor and respect of others, resulting in family disgrace) or inducing stigma and embarrassment so that they may not be willing to talk with 'outsiders' about the challenging or disturbing behaviors of their children with LD. Because of 'saving face', the Chinese parents may exert a high self-control and avoid disclosing the illness or misfortune to the 'outsiders' (Li-Tsang, Yau & Yuen, 2001). This may result in their being reluctant to seek help or share with others, and health professionals, about their difficulties in caregiving (Chien et al., 2007). Health professionals should explore these parents' 'hidden' and 'unmet' health needs, encourage them to openly express these needs, and then offer them culture-specific and appropriate advices on caregiving.

Finally, female or mothers in both Chinese and Western culture (Pinquart & Sorensen 2006), mostly are the primary carers for children with chronic conditions. The mothers in this study reported much more difficulties in child care and accentuated feelings of abandonment and social discrimination than those fathers and they perceived that they themselves received inadequate support from their spouse or other family members. Female carers who usually express high levels of distress and helplessness, should be much concerned with their psychosocial well-being (Saloviita et al., 2003); and at the earliest moment, health professionals should provide additional psychosocial support and counseling for them to prevent marital disharmony and impairments of family relationships and functioning.

Limitations of the Study

There were a few limitations in the study. The research was conducted in a two small mental health centers in which the parental carers indicated similar levels of secondary education and socio-economic backgrounds. On one hand, they might present much a lot of similarities in their beliefs and perceptions about their caregiving and health needs; but on the other hand, there could be different types of parental needs in others with diverse socio-demographic backgrounds. A more comprehensive coverage of parents or carers from different districts and backgrounds should be recruited in future study to fully understand the parental health needs in caring for a child with LD. In addition, children with different types of developmental and learning problems should be explored and compared to fully answer the parental health needs in specialized care for these children. In addition, family carers might have specific sets of health needs or concerns at different stages and symptom severities of LD. Therefore, further research on parents' education and support needs in terms of illness type or severity should be considered.

Last, the use of semi-structured interview only for data collection, and tap-recording of the interviews, might also have made the researcher not able to validate or confirm the results and the parents be self-conscious and desirably respond to interview questions, respectively. Methodological triangulation using different data collection methods, such as field observation and personal diary, can be considered to address the credibility and dependability of the findings in a qualitative research (Burns & Grove, 2010).

Conclusion

The findings of this study indicate a few major health educational needs of parents in taking care of a child with learning disability that has been underestimated by mental health and educational service providers. Information about the illness, adequate social support and appropriate and accessible family services should be provided for these parents to provide effective care for their child with LD. To facilitate effective parenting, specific and focused needs assessment and education should be provided to address parental caregiving and associated health needs in the realms of bio-psychosocial and cultural domains. Further research are recommended to explore family carers' holistic health needs and coping ability in caregiving, in family populations with diverse socio-economic and cultural backgrounds in Chinese and Asian countries.

References

American Psychiatric Association. (2000). *Diagnostic and Statistical Manual of Mental Disorders, 4th Text Revised Version* (DSM IV-TR). Washington, DC: The author.

Antshel, K. M. & Joseph, G. R. (2006). Maternal stress in nonverbal learning disorder: A comparison with reading disorder. *Journal of Learning Disabilities, 39,* 194-207.

Azar, M. & Badr, L. K. (2006). The adaptation of mothers of children with intellectual disability in Lebanon. *Journal of Transcultural Nursing, 17*, 375-380.

Bowen, G. A. (2008). Naturalistic inquiry and the saturation concept: A research note. *Qualitative Research, 8*, 137-152.

Bull, C. & Whelan, T. (2006). Parental schemata in the management of children with attention deficit-hyperactivity disorder. *Qualitative Health Research, 16*, 664-678.

Burns, N. & Grove, S. K. (2010). U*nderstanding nursing research: Building an evidence-based practice* (5th ed.). St. Louis, MO: Saunders Elsevier.

Buschgens, C., van Aken, M., Swinkels, S., Altin, M., Fliers, E., Rommelese, N., et al. (2008). Differential family and peer environmental factors are related to severity and co-morbidity in children with ADHD. *Journal of Neural Transmission, 115*, 177-186.

Chan, C. W. (2008). Overview of specific learning disabilities/dyslexia developments over the last decade in Hong Kong. *Hong Kong Journal of Paediatrics, 13*, 196-202.

Chan, C. W., Ho, C. S. H., Tsang, S. M., Lee, S. H. & Chung, K. K. H. (2008). Estimating incidence of developmental dyslexia in Hong Kong: What differences do different criteria make? *Australian Journal of Learning Difficulties, 13*, 1-16.

Chang, M. Y. & Hsu, L. L. (2007). The perceptions of Taiwanese families who have children with learning disability. *Journal of Clinical Nursing, 16,* 2349-2356.

Chien, W. T., Chan, W. C. S. & Morrissey, J. (2007). The perceived burden among Chinese family caregivers of people with schizophrenia. *Journal of Clinical Nursing, 16*, 1151-1161.

Chien, W. T. & Lee, Y. M. I. (2013). An exploratory study of parents' perceived educational needs in parenting a child with learning disabilities. *Asian Nursing Research*, *7*(1), 16-25.

Chien, W. T., Norman, I. & Thompson, D. R. (2006). Perceived benefits and difficulties experienced in a mutual support group for family carers of people with schizophrenia. *Qualitative Health Research, 16*, 962-981.

Crnic, K. A., Gaze, C. & Hoffman, C. (2005). Cumulative parenting stress across the preschool period: relations to maternal parenting and child behavior at age 5. *Infant and Child Development, 14*, 117-132.

Denzin, N. K. & Lincoln Y. S. (2005). *The Sage handbook of qualitative research* (3rd ed.). London, UK: Sage Publications.

Elder, J. H. (2001). A follow-up study of beliefs held by parents of children with pervasive developmental delay. *Journal of Child and Adolescent Psychiatric Nursing, 14*, 55-60.

Gannon, S. & McGilloway, S. (2009). Children's attitudes toward their peers with Down Syndrome in schools in rural Ireland: An exploratory study. *European Journal of Special Needs Education, 24*, 445-463.

Gilstrap L. (2004). A missing link in suggestibility research: What is known about the behavior of field interviewers in unstructured interviews with young children? *Journal of Experimental Psychology: Applied, 10, 13-24.*

Graneheim, U. H. & Lundman, B. (2004). Qualitative content analysis in nursing research: Concepts, procedures and measures to achieve trustworthiness. *Nurse Education Today, 24*, 105-112.

Griffiths, P., Bennett, J. & Smith, E. (2008). The size, extent and nature of the learning disability nursing research base: A systematic scoping review. *International Journal of Nursing Studies, 46*, 490-507.

Harrison, C. & Sofronoff, K. (2002). ADHD and parental psychological distress: Role of demographics, child behavioral characteristics, and parental cognitions. *Journal of American Academy of Child & Adolescent Psychiatry, 41*, 703-711.

Heiman, T. (2002). Parents of children with disabilities: Resilience, coping, and future expectations. *Journal of Developmental and Physical Disabilities, 14*, 159-171.

Hill, C. & Rose, J. (2009). Parenting stress in mothers of adults with an intellectual disability: Parental cognitions in relation to child characteristics and family support. *Journal of Intellectual Disability Research, 49*, 405-417.

Ho, C., Chien, W. T. & Wang, L. Q. (2011). Parents' experiences of caring for a child with attention deficit hyperactivity disorder: An exploratory study. *Contemporary Nurse, 40*, 41-56.

Hong Kong Association of Specific Learning Disabilities. (2010). *Parents' Manual.* Retrieved 10 December 2010, from http://www.asld.org.hk/.

Karande, S. & Kulkarni, S. (2009). Quality of life of parents of children with newly diagnosed specific learning disability. *Journal of Postgraduate Medicine, 55*, 97-103.

Karande, S., Mehta, V. & Kulkarni, M. (2007). Impact of an education program on parental knowledge of specific learning disability. *Indian Journal of Medical Sciences, 61*, 308-406.

Keller, D. & Honig, A. S. (2004). Maternal and paternal stress in families with school-aged children with disabilities. *American Journal of Orthopsychiatry, 74,* 337–348.

Kendall, J., Leo, M. C., Perrin, N. & Hatton, D. (2005). Modeling ADHD child and family relationships. *Western Journal of Nursing Research, 27*, 500-518.

Kenny, K. & McGilloway, S. (2007). Caring for children with learning disabilities: An exploratory study of parental strain and coping. *British Journal of Learning Disabilities, 35*, 221-228.

Lam, C. (2005). Services for developmental dyslexia in Hong Kong. *Hong Kong Journal of Paediatrics, 10*, 149-152.

Lazarus, R. S. (1991). *Emotion and adaptation*. New York: Oxford University Press.

Lazarus, R. S. & Folkman, S. (1984). *Stress, appraisal and coping*. New York: Springer.

Li-Tsang, W. P. C., Yau, K. S. M. & Yuen, H. K. (2001). Success in parenting children with developmental disabilities: Some characteristics, attitudes and adaptive coping skills. *British Journal of Developmental Disabilities, 47*, 61-71.

Little, L. (2002). Differences in stress and coping for mothers and fathers of children with Asperger's syndrome and nonverbal learning disorders. *Pediatric Nursing, 28*, 582-583.

Little, L. & Clark, R. R. (2006). Wonders and worries of parenting a child with Asperger syndrome and nonverbal learning disorder MCN. *The American Journal of Maternal/Child Nursing, 31*, 39-44.

Morse, J. M. (2000). Determining sample size. *Qualitative Health Research, 10*, 3-5.

Munhall, P. L., 2000. *Qualitative research proposals and reports: A guide*. Sudbury, MA: Jones and Bartlett.

National Institute for Health and Clinical Excellence. (2008). *NICE clinical guideline 72 - Diagnosis and management of ADHD in children, young people and adults*. London, UK: National Collaborating Centre for Mental Health.

Ngan Keung, I. W. L. (2008). Public awareness, community services and parent support. *Hong Kong Journal of Paediatrics, 13*, 213-217.

Phetrasuwan, S. & Miles, M. S. (2009). Parenting stress in mothers of children with autism spectrum disorders. *Journal for Specialists in Paediatric Nursing, 14*, 157-165.

Pinquart, M. & Sorensen, S. (2006). Gender differences in caregiver stressors, social resources, and health: An updated meta-analysis. *Journal of Gerontology Series B: Psychological Sciences & Social Sciences, 61*, 33-45.

Rayner, M. & Moore, S. (2007). Stress and ameliorating factors among families with a seriously ill or disabled child. *Journal of Applied Psychology, 3*, 86-93.

Saloviita, T., Italinna, M. & Leinonen, E. (2003). Explaining the parental stress of fathers and mothers caring for a child with intellectual disability: A double ABCX model. *Journal of Intellectual Disability, 47*, 300-312.

Smythe, I., Everatt, J. & Salter, R. (2003). *The international book of dyslexia: A guide to practice and resources*. Edinburgh, UK: Wiley-Blackwell.

Waggoner, K. & Wilgosh, L. (1990). Concerns of families of children with learning disabilities. *Journal of Learning Disabilities, 23*, 97-113.

In: Caregivers
Editor: Adrienne Lloyd
ISBN: 978-1-63483-909-9

Chapter 5

PERCEPTION AND ATTITUDE OF CAREGIVERS: IMPLICATION FOR CHILDHOOD SEXUAL ABUSE DISCLOSURE

Adebunmi Oyebisi Alade*
Department of Guidance and Counselling
University of Ibadan, Ibadan, Nigeria

ABSTRACT

Over recent years, the number of reported cases of sexual abuse in children has increased with new and bizarre cases every day, most especially in Nigeria. However, the true prevalence is difficult to ascertain because it is a crime that flourishes in secrecy. This is promoted by the unrelenting perpetrator as well as victims' family members who wish to maintain and protect the family dignity and honour to avoid stigmatization. Disclosure is a delicate and sensitive process which is influenced by several factors, including implicit or explicit pressure for secrecy, feelings of guilt, shame, fear of negative consequences and/or embarrassment.

Although, sexual abuse of children provokes reactions of indignation and incomprehensibility in all cultures, the perception and attitudes of caregivers could affect reporting of sexual abuse, prosecution of perpetrators, and provision of clinical services. The nature and quality of support and protection from caregivers provides an effective platform for quick recovery and improvement in mental health and social functioning of victims. Unfortunately, not all caregivers are supportive of survivors; instead, disclosure of childhood sexual abuse is often met with disbelief, anger, or rejection which leaves victim feeling isolated and unworthy.

This paper therefore, aims at improving the understanding on disclosure trends, impacts, and factors that may inhibit or motivate children to disclose sexual abuse experience(s).

Keywords: attitude, caregivers, childhood sexual abuse, disclosure, perception

* aladebunmi2008@yahoo.com; 0802-390-6266; 0814-626-7027.

INTRODUCTION

Child sexual abuse (CSA) is a complex social problem which has become increasingly frequent globally; with its attendant wide range of negative psychosocial outcomes and consequences throughout childhood and into adulthood for both child victims and their families. The range of mental health outcomes associated with child sexual abuse is as broad and varied as the nature of the abuse situations although the extent and severity of these differ for each individual. Researchers have identified a multitude of negative psychological outcomes of child sexual abuse experiences. These include both short and long term consequences such as withdrawn behaviours, nightmares, emotional stress, posttraumatic stress disorder, anxiety, depression and low self-esteem, inappropriate sexualized behaviour and difficulty with peer relationships (Alade, 2015; Cutajar et al., 2010; Banyard, Williams & Siegal, 2001; Mullen, Martin, Anderson, Romans & Herbison, 1993; Mullens, Martin, Anderson, Romans & Herbison, 1996).

DEFINITION AND PREVALENCE OF SEXUAL ABUSE

Child sexual abuse in the broadest sense encompasses not only the inappropriate touching of children but also using children in sexual trafficking, pornography, and prostitution. The Royal College of Psychiatrists (2012) defined sexual abuse of children as sexually interfering with or assaulting a child. According to Browne and Finkelhor (1996) there are two overlapping but distinguishable types of interaction in defining childhood sexual abuse: (a) forced or coerced sexual behaviour imposed on a child, and (b) sexual activity between a child and a much older person, whether or not obvious coercion is involved (which connotes a common definition of "much older" is 5 or more years).

A variety of specific sexual activities have been considered to be childhood sexual abuse (intercourse, oral-genital contact, attempted intercourse, fondling of genitals (directly or through clothing), exhibitionism or exposing children to adult sexual activity or pornography, and the use of a child for prostitution or pornography including the grooming and sexual abuse of children via technology and the internet. With the recent technological advancement and establishment of numerous social interaction and networking sites the internet provides an opportunity for children to be seduced by perpetrators into future abuse while they are online even within their own homes (Child Exploitation and Online Protection (CEOP) 2012; Byron, 2010; Livingstone, Haddon, Gorzig & Olafsson, 2010; Putnam, 2003). Although, there is still a general lack of societal consensus regarding activities that constitute sexual abuse as well as discrepancies in age limits, in sum for research purposes definitions of CSA simply requires two elements; (1) sexual activities (contact and noncontact) involving a child and (2) an "abusive condition" based on the abuser (large age gap, position of authority or caretaker, coercion or force).

With reported definitional and methodological differences between studies on the phenomenon of child sexual abuse, it suggests that reliable estimates of prevalence are difficult to establish. Given these difficulties, it is likely that published statistics on the prevalence of child sexual abuse are underestimates of the true rate of occurrence of the problem. Recent international studies reported that between 8 - 31 per cent of girls and 3-17 per cent of boys experience childhood sexual abuse (Finkelhor, 2014; Barth, Bermetz, Heim, Trelle & Tonia, 2013).

Disclosure of Sexual Abuse

It is widely accepted that the true incidence of childhood sexual abuse is significantly higher because it is perpetrated in private, but unfortunately, many cases are neither disclosed by victims nor detected and reported by other persons. It is estimated that less than one in four CSA victims disclose to someone immediately following the abuse (Paine & Hansen, 2002). Disclosure refers to the way children, young people or adults let other people know they are being or have been sexually abused. It refers to "the telling of abuse," regardless of the specific individual (formal or informal network) to whom the victim discloses (Lovett, 2004; Ullman, 2003).

Forms of Disclosure

Disclosures of sexual abuse can occur in different forms. These are accidental and purposeful disclosure. Mian, Wehrspann, Klajner-Diamond, Le Baron and Winder (1986) defined purposeful disclosure as an intentional and deliberate revelation of the abuse with clear intent of revealing its existence. Purposeful disclosures connotes that the victim of the sexual abuse decided to tell an outsider who may or may not be the victim's immediate family member. Either way, it leads to the parent's finding out. Once the decision to disclose the abuse is decided, the victim must determine in whom she should confide. On the other hand, accidental disclosure is a statement made without forethought or intent to reveal the abusive relationship. Accidental disclosures are revealed through discovery of the act itself or through clues leading to the sexual behavior. This type of disclosure is considered accidental because no one intended to tell of the abuse or have people discover that the abuse was occurring. Accidental disclosure may occur when a physical symptom is detected or when a child displays some behavioural or emotional symptom (Shackel, 2009).

Additionally, disclosure could be prompted or elicited (Jones, 2000; Paine & Hansen, 2002; Hershkowitz, Lanes & Lamb, 2007). This refers to disclosures that are assisted by other people and precipitant disclosure occurs when an event prompts or triggers a memory of the abuse (Campis et al. 1993). Allnock and Miller (2013) reported that in a qualitative study of disclosure among 60 young men and women in the United Kingdom eight forms of disclosure were discovered. These include direct, indirect verbal, partial verbal, accidental direct/verbal, prompted, non-verbal/behavioural, retracted and assisted. Partial disclosures were characterized by minimization of the abuse, disclosing abuse of another person or disclosing other forms of abuse such as physical assault. While on the other hand, prompted disclosures were made in response to a direct inquiry about abuse while assisted disclosures involved a young person disclosing to another young person with the help of a friend. Children use a variety of techniques to disclose including direct or ambiguous verbal statements and non-verbal disclosure in the form of writing letters, re-enacting abuse type situations or drawing pictures for adults.

MODELS OF DISCLOSURE

The conceptualization of disclosure has received growing attention has it has been conceived as an event or as a continuum or process (Summit et al. 1983; Furniss, 1990; Bussey & Grimbeek, 1995; Goodman-Brown, Edelstien, Goodman, Jones & Gordon, 2003; Alaggia, 2004; Staller & Nelson-Gardell, 2005). However, most work on the sequence or stages of disclosure emanates from Summit (1983) who first proposed a linear model identifying the successive phases of the disclosure process known as the Child Sexual Abuse Accommodation Syndrome to explain how children disclose and why they may be reluctant to do so. Summit's model included five components. The first two components are identified as fundamental to the occurrence of sexual abuse while others are noted to be complex sequential contingencies that may vary (Summit, 1983). These components are:

1. *Secrecy* (keeping the abuse secret): In most cases sexual abuse occurs only when the child is alone with the offending adult. Regardless of the means by which the perpetrator invokes the child to keep the abuse secret, secrecy inherently conveys to the child that the abuse is something bad and dangerous. Perpetrators foretell that disclosure will result in dreadful outcomes for the victim, loved ones, and the perpetrator. Hence, the message imparted to the child is, ''Maintaining a lie to keep the secret is the ultimate virtue, while telling the truth would be the greatest sin'' (Summit, 1983).
2. *Helplessness* (feeling of powerlessness to stop or communicate the abuse): The expectation of others that children will self-protect and immediately disclose ''ignores the basic subordination and helplessness of children within authoritarian relationships'' (Summit, 1983). They are expected to be obedient, even affectionate, with adults responsible for their care.
3. *Entrapment or accommodation* (learning to accept and accommodate the sexual abuse as a reality): Faced with a seemingly inescapable situation in which the child feels helpless, learning to accommodate to the sexual abuse is the only healthy alternative available. The means by which children accommodate include, but are not limited to, assuming personal responsibility for the abuse, adopting the distorted beliefs of the perpetrator, dissociating, and suppressing or repressing memories of the abuse.
4. *Delayed (*conflicted and unconvincing disclosure): Most victims of ongoing abuse never disclose their victimization (Summit, 1983). When they do, delayed disclosure is the norm. The delayed and conflicted manner in which victims disclose casts doubt on their credibility.
5. *Retraction* (disclosing abuse and subsequent retracting): During the aftermath of disclosure, the child's anticipated fears regarding disclosure often become reality. Faced with others disbelief, lack of support, and the upheaval following disclosure, the child may retract the allegation of abuse in an attempt to undo the damage and restore equilibrium. Summit theorized that a child accommodates to the abuse and does not disclose as a means of coping. While this model has been endorsed by many clinicians (Carnes, Wilson, Nelson-Gardell & Ogassa, 2001; McElvaney, 2013) research suggests that there is little empirical evidence to support the tenets of the

model beyond the silence/secrecy stage (London, Bruck, Ceci & Shuman, 2005). Building on Summit's work, Furniss (1991) identified external and internal factors that contributed to the abuse being kept a secret.

Social Exchange Model of Disclosure

Exchange theories are based on the guiding premise that "individuals pursue those social relationships and interactions based on perceptions of rewards and costs. By implication those in which they get the best payoffs or the greatest reward for the least cost" (Leonard, 1996). Leonard (1996) provided an analysis of the Child Sexual Abuse Accommodation Syndrome (Summit, 1983) from the perspective of social exchange theory. Conversely, individuals avoid exchange relations that are high in cost to them. The potential for the use or abuse of power is intrinsic to the exchange perspective (Leonard, 1996).

In this vein, Leonard noted that Blau (1964) proposed definition of power be expanded to read that "it is the ability of persons or groups to impose their will on others despite resistance through deterrence either in the forms of withholding regularly supplied rewards or in the form of punishment, both being negative sanctions" (Blau, 1964). Applying principles of cost and rewards to each of the five components of the CSA Accommodation Syndrome, Leonard attempts to demonstrate that each component reflects the least unprofitable of the limited options child victims perceive are available. This theory was extended to perpetrators and members of the victim's family. The application of exchange theory to one component of the CSA Accommodation Syndrome (i.e., entrapment and accommodation) is offered to illustrate that repeated sexual abuse without intervention, the child victim holds little hope for rescue or a timely end to the abuse (entrapment). From the perspective of exchange-equity theory, an individual in an inequitable relationship with another grows increasingly distressed as the inequity mounts. "In order to reduce the distress, an individual can restore actual equity (rarely an option for a child in an abusive dyad) or psychological equity" (Leonard, 1996). Psychological equity is achieved by distorting reality in order to convince themselves that the treatment they are receiving is deserved (accommodation). Research has demonstrated that under the right conditions, both "exploiters" and their victims are capable of convincing themselves that even the most inequitable exchanges are fair (Leonard, 1996; Walster, 1978; Walster, Walster & Berscheid, 1978). The perpetrator conveys the notion to the child that being good means being available and compliant. "Frequently, there is an implicit or explicit promise of reward to the child for being 'good,' such as the preservation of the home, and/or the protection of siblings from sexual abuse" (Leonard, 1996).

Social–Cognitive Model

Bussey and Grimbeek (1995) proposed a dynamic and interactive model whereby disclosure was multi-determined. The model posits that there are four socio-cognitive determinants of disclosure: attention; retention; production; and motivation. They noted that these four component processes were initially proposed by Bandura to account for children's observational learning as bystanders. This model of disclosure purports that "the course of disclosure will vary according to children's cognitive capabilities, social experience, and the particular situation in which they find themselves'' (Bussey & Grimbeek, 1995). The model offers a theoretical basis for research findings that reveal lower rates of disclosure among older children. From a cognitive perspective, older children are better able to report their abuse due to increased attentional, retentional, and production skills. However, with increased cognitive abilities and social experience, children become more aware of the costs and benefits of disclosure. For these reasons, it is anticipated that children's disclosure will be more self-regulated as they mature (Bussey & Grimbeek, 1995).

Disclosure may be inhibited when children ''have not paid sufficient attention to the event (attention processes), they are unable to remember it in sufficient detail (retention processes), they are unable to adequately communicate about the event (production processes), or they are unwilling to report it (motivation processes)'' (Bussey & Grimbeek, 1995). They noted that disclosure varied according to a child's cognitive capacity and their experience of the world.

Goodman-Brown et al. (2003) developed a model whereby self-blame, fears of the consequence of telling, or others reactions, were key factors influencing delays in disclosure. In studying the experiences of disclosure among 34 female adolescents, Staller and Nelson-Gardell (2005) proposed a three staged framework that includes: the self (coming to terms with feelings of abuse) recipient selection and reaction (selecting how and when to tell and coping with the reaction) and consideration of consequence to explain the disclosure process. According to Hunter (2011) it is important to include the person to whom the disclosure is made in any model of disclosure because telling a friend, family members and police are very different experiences. These models contribute to the literature by emphasizing that disclosure is not linear and sequential but rather a dynamic and interactive process that is influenced by how children receive and process information about the abuse and the abuser and make decisions about whom they tell.

Rates of Disclosure

Studies have shown that victims frequently either fail to disclose the abuse or delay disclosure for years (Ullman, 2003; Martin & Silverstone, 2013). In a national survey of adult men and women, Finkelhor, Hotaling, Lewis, and Smith (1990) noted that 33% of women and 42% of men never disclosed their abuse experience to anyone. Banyard, Arnold, and Smith (2000) reported that 72% of women disclosed their CSA experiences, but 47% of those who disclosed did not disclose to anyone for 5 years or more following the abuse (Ullman, 2003). Allagia and Kirshenbaum (2005) reported that the latency of disclosure indicates delays ranging from 3 to 18 years. In a community sample involving 3,000 women Mullen, Martin, Anderson, Romans-Clarkson, and Herbison (1993) specifically noted delays in disclosure and found that 37% of the victims disclosed within the first year following the abuse, 10% disclosed 1-10 years after, 24% disclosed beyond 10 years, and 28% had never disclosed. London, Bruck, Ceci, and Shuman (2005) noted disclosure rates among college samples ranged from 24% to 38%. Similarly, Arata (1998) found in a sample of college women, that only one third of victims disclosed at the time of the abuse and, of those who disclosed, 40% of the victims told only one person. In contrast, Kellogg and Hutson (1995) reported that 85% of the young adult victims in their study had disclosed, although the timing of the disclosure was not specified. Studies of adults have found delays of up to 50 years (McElvaney, 2002). Lamb and Edgar-Smith (1994) found that the mean age for first disclosure was 18 years, while the mean age of abuse onset for those in the sample was 8 years, resulting in an average delay of 10 years in their sample of adults. In the Collings, Griffiths and Kumalo (2005) study of children who had experienced penetrative abuse, 47% had reported the abuse within 72 hours, 31% from 72 hours to one month after the abuse, and 22% more than a month after the abuse. However, Smith et al. (2000) estimated that 48% of young women in their survey had told no one for more than five years after the event. As such, child sexual abuse incident rates, only represent the tip of the iceberg as a great proportion of children delay disclosure or refuse to do so at all (London, Bruck, Ceci & Shuman, 2007).

Factors Inhibiting Disclosure

Some motivational factors have been identified which make some children reluctant to disclose sexual abuse experience. Indeed, research has shown tremendous individual differences in a child's capacity to evoke events, depending on their gender, age, as well as the nature of the child-perpetrator relationship (Pipe, Lamb, Orbach & Cederborg, 2007).

Child's Gender

Consistently gender differences have been reported in the prevalence rates of child sexual abuse. This may be due to higher instances of sexual abuse among girls than boys. However, boys have been found to have more reluctant attitude towards disclosing their sexual abuse experiences (Romano & De Luca, 2001). Indeed, boys in general seem more reluctant than girls to disclose information regarding sexual abuse (Ghetti & Goodman, 2001). Girls also tend to provide more detailed account of abuse than boys (Lamb & Garretson, 2003). According to Hershkowitz et al. (2007) older boys make fewer allegations when the sexual abuse is perpetrated by a parent or parent-figure as compared to girls. This difference was not found in cases of physical abuse, demonstrating the important impact of a child's gender, age, and the victim perpetrator relationship especially in cases of child sexual abuse disclosure.

Child's Age

Although age has a significant impact on the quantity of information revealed by children at disclosure, findings differ on the direction of the impact. For instance Lamb, Malloy and Rooy (2011) argued that age in itself does not determine children's ability to recount personal traumatic experience(s) but rather serves to summarize the influence of a number of interrelated psychological factors (i.e., cognitive or emotional variables such as language and memory capacity. Young children as compared to adults have more idiosyncratic and limited vocabularies (e.g., interpret words concretely), and are less effective in coping with misunderstandings. Moreover, they usually have not developed the concept of time (Orbach & Lamb, 2007). Although individual differences exist, language development and communication skills tend to increase and solidify over time, they also seem to be prerequisites for children to fully remember and recount them to others (Lamb, Malloy & Rooy, 2011).

Furthermore, a meta-analysis of studies on children's memories revealed that age is the most important determinant of children's memory capacity. Basically, children are gradually able to remember their experiences for longer and longer periods of time. How well they remember an event depends at least partly on how well they understood the incident and can associate it to other experiences in their memory (i.e., making links with past experiences). Older children may, therefore, be better at encoding new events because they tend to better understand and process the event based on having more knowledge and past experiences. This knowledge is used to generate cues to link the event with other experiences and may therefore facilitate retrieval and thus lead to more detailed disclosures (Lamb, Malloy & Rooy, 2011). According to Lamb, Hershkowitz, Orbach, and Esplin (2008) younger children may misunderstand the abuse itself, thereby failing to disclose all pertinent information. Preschoolers may also lack the cognitive, communicative and emotional ability to understand and describe their abuse experiences (Lamb et al., 2008). However, Goodman-Brown, Edelstein, Goodman, Jones and Gordon (2003) showed that older children more often delay sexual abuse disclosure because they may feel more responsible for the incident and believe they could have prevented the abuse and, as a result, try to keep it secret. Moreover, adolescents may be more willing to withhold information than younger children because of their amplified awareness of the consequences of disclosure. Or, perhaps some of the younger non-disclosing children later decide to disclose. Therefore it is pertinent to conceptualize what exactly is meant where the impact of children's age during child sexual abuse disclosure is considered.

Child-Perpetrator Relationship

There is a tendency for children of all ages to have higher non-disclosure rates when the suspect is a member of their immediate family. Children may be motivated to withhold information because they have been pressured to remain silent or wish to protect familial suspects, especially caregivers on whom they are dependent (Hershkowitz et al., 2007; Paine & Hansen, 2002; Pipe et al., 2007; Summit, 1983). Hershkowitz et al. (2007) found that children who were suspected victims of parental abuse provided proportionally fewer informative and more uninformative responses (e.g., omission, "don't know," "don't want to talk," "don't remember") leading to fewer details per response, than suspected victims of non-parental abuse. There is a tendency for children of all ages to have higher non-disclosure rates when the suspect is an immediate family member. Hershkowitz, Lanes, and Lamb(2007) assessed sexual abuse disclosure by extra-familial perpetrators and proposed that children were more likely to delay disclosure (ranging from one week to two years) in more severe cases involving intrusive sexual acts (e.g., penetration) and multiple incidents as opposed to single incidents involving non-intrusive acts (e.g., touching over the clothes). Additional, results indicated that it is more difficult for children severely abused by a familiar perpetrator on multiple occasions to confess spontaneously than it is for children abused only once by a complete stranger (e.g., cases of exhibitionism). In addition, children more often expressed fear or shame when the perpetrators were familiar (78%), the abuse was serious (83%) or repeated (79%). As a result, feelings of distress could have a direct impact on a child's degree of cooperation even when they decide to disclose sexual abuse experiences. Overall, the results indicate that children who suffer severe and frequent sexual abuse, especially by people who they know, tend to disclose belatedly, hesitantly, and indirectly.

Reasons for Non- disclosure

According to Ullman (2003) not disclosing sexual abuse occurrence has many deleterious effects for victims including inability to stop further abuse and not receiving therapeutic interventions. Clearly, significant delays in disclosing sexual abuse inhibit any attempt to reach an accurate estimate of the extent of the problem of child sexual abuse in society. Malhotra and Biwas (2005) reported that the current societal attitudes and practices toward children and societal tolerance towards abuse can provide a fertile environment for child sexual abuse. This tolerance is expressed through the denial of the existence or pervasiveness of child sexual abuse and the minimization or outright denial of the harmful effects of childhood sexual abuse. Throughout history, backlash movements, denial, and minimization of child sexual abuse survive because of strong emotional reactions which result in a protective, reflexive denial of child sexual abuse awareness. Lindblom and Carlsson (2001) reported that cognitive dissonance is an alternative explanation for this reflexive denial in which the society is uncomfortable with believing atrocities exist such as the high prevalence rate of child sexual abuse. Societal believing also influences victims' perceptions of whether it is safe to disclose abuse and the will to actually disclose (Somer & Szwarcberg, 2001).

Furthermore, believing victims' disclosures is related to providing positive social support, which in turn, is strongly related to better health outcomes for victims (Ullman & Filipas, 2005). Goodman- Brown, Edelstein, Goodman, Jones and Gordon (2003) averred that fear of not being believed by parents or caregiver is a major deterrent against sexual abuse disclosure. Ullman (2003) opined that not being believed has negative psychological and physiological health effects on the victim. Other literature suggested that adolescents may not disclose their experiences due to fear of social stigmatization (Ahrens, Campbell, Ternier – Thames, Wasco & Sefl, 2007; Banyard, Moynihan, Walsh, Cohn & Ward, 2010) acceptance of rape myths (Frese, Moya & Megías, 2004; Hillenbrand – Gunn, Heppner, Mauch & Park, 2010) and internalized blame patterns (Banyard et al., 2010; Barter, 2009; Daignault & Hebert, 2009). Consequently, many adolescents who experience sexual abuse may be too afraid of the social and disciplinary consequences imposed upon them by friends and parents respectively. In a study conducted by Livingston, Hequembourg, Testsa, and Van-Ziletamson (2007) many victims claimed they could not report their abuse because they had lied to their parents about the party where the incident occurred, and thus, feared disciplinary consequences.

There are other documented factors that influence a victim's decision not to disclose. Jensen et al. (2005) reported that many disclosures are determined by prompts from others and open opportunities to talk. They further noted that many victims found it difficult to disclose because of a lack of suitable private situations and that disclosure was easier when child sexual abuse was addressed (Jensen et al., 2005). Consequently, cultural factors and family dynamics can be inhibiting factors to disclosure by depriving child sexual abuse victims of such open opportunities to talk. For example, Allagia and Kirshenbaum (2005) reported that "disclosure may be inhibited in families whose cultures hold taboos and negative attitudes about sexuality and that place a high premium on preservation of family. Other noted reasons for non-disclosure are embarrassment and shame, fear of negative reactions and consequences, protecting others, and threats made by the abuser (Ullman, 2003). Ultimately, a victim's decision to disclose or not to disclose has the potential to affect mental health outcomes of child sexual abuse which has been associated with decreased distress and physical symptoms. Generally, an abused child is reluctant to tell anyone about the experiences. Therefore, the response of the confidant, in the event that the child decides to disclose, is very important. If the caregiver is impatient or judgmental, it may make the abuse have more profound negative effects on the child, making the child have feelings of guilt as if it were the victim's fault the abuse happened.

Caregivers Attitude and Perception of Sexual Abuse Disclosure

Dealing with disclosure of sexual abuse is both complex and challenging for parents. This is because disclosure and learning of a one-off or ongoing sexual abuse of child is likely to be an intense, upsetting, unexpected and confusing event. This understandably could leads to psychological distress in parents manifested in a variety of ways. There is a myriad of both positive and negative caregiver reactions to CSA disclosures. The disclosure may trigger feelings of failure for some parents (Hebert, Daigneault, Collin-Vezina & Cyr, 2007). A child's disclosure may trigger past sexual trauma of the mother, further confirming the need for support and counseling to help her cope with the consequences of disclosure (Hebert et al., 2007). Reported positive reactions include belief, validation, not being blamed, protectiveness, listening, willingness to talk about the effects of the abuse, accepting attitude, as well as assuring the child that the abuse will not reoccur (instrumental support). Conversely, commonly reported negative reactions include disbelief, blame, ignoring the victim (refusing to talk), minimization, parental rejection, neglect, indifference, hostility, avoidance, punishment, stigma, accusation of lying, and a lack of decisive steps to stop the abuse (Ullman, 2003).

Most often disclosure is met with disbelief, anger, or rejection which leaves a child feeling isolated, unnoticed and unsure. Children don't disclose because they are afraid of the consequences to themselves and others, they feel ashamed or in some way responsible for the abuse, they are unsure whether an abuse has occurred, or they do not know where to turn to for help. Children therefore make calculated decisions about disclosing; they consider who they will tell, whether they will be believed and how much detail they should provide. Literature suggests that the reactions a victim receives following disclosure of abuse may directly affect the psychological outcomes associated with the abuse and the disclosure (Lovett, 2004; Ullman, 2003). Many adult CSA survivors indicated that their childhood sexual abuse disclosures were met with negative reactions such as blame or encouraging secrecy, and many times the abuse did not end following disclosure. For example, in a study of 83 confirmed cases of CSA records showed that in 20 of the 83 cases the confidant did not report the abuse to anyone following the victim's disclosure (Paine & Hansen, 2002). Furthermore, Jensen et al. (2005) reported that in a sample of 22 CSA victims and their families most people to whom the victims disclosed initially responded with shock and looked for alternative explanations for why the child was indicating abuse (Ullman, 2003). Ullman (2003) reported that a variety of studies have documented a wide range of negative reactions to CSA disclosures as well as the significant adverse effects of negative reactions on psychosocial adjustment and psychological health. Support and protection from the caregiver provides the child an effective platform for quick recovery and improvement in mental health and social functioning (Lovett, 2004). Nonetheless, not all caregivers are supportive of survivors; recent research findings, instead, showed that incidents of CSA have debilitating psychological impact on survivors' caregivers which impair their parental functioning (Bolan & Lamb, 2004).

The cognitive and emotional responses from parents are usually similar to that of the victims. Caregivers or parents may sometimes experience guilt about the sexual abuse occurring without their being able to protect the victim. Generalized fear about things such as leaving the house and leaving their children alone, grief over the experiences their child has gone through, as well as a feeling of loss surrounding their child's innocence pervade the parent's life. Mothers especially struggled with self-esteem issues, feeling as though they were not a good mother (Womack, Miller & Lassiter, 1999). Powerlessness in the abuse's occurring is often felt as a result of not being able to change the past and protect their child.

Often times, the caregivers' responses appear to progress through the stages of grief. The grief is centered on the loss of their feelings of safety and control within their family home, According to Kubler-Ross (1969), the stages of grief consist of denial, anger, bargaining, depression, and finally acceptance. During the denial stage, caregivers are in disbelief that the sexual abuse occurred. The denial was followed by anger at themselves, the perpetrators, and/or even the victims for the abuse and the subsequent changes which the abuse precipitated. Bargaining occurred when mothers try to reason with themselves or a supreme being, such as God, in an attempt to either gain back time or make things right for the victim. After this point, depression seemed to set in and the non-offending parents had difficulty in proceeding with their daily life. Lastly, these caregivers came to terms with the sexual abuse and began to take action to protect their children from future abuse situations.

For non-offending parents, their initial responses of shock and denial transitioned into anger, bargaining, depression, and finally acceptance of the abuse. These feelings of loss, confusion, and conflict can occur within the family, focusing on the victims, perpetrators, and extended family members for their support or lack of support following the abuse disclosure. These feelings may also take place with people who were considered outside of the family such as therapists, police officers, and judges who may have conflicting ideas of what action the parents should have taken during the abuse or should have taken following the disclosure (Womack, Miller & Lassiter, 1999).

Research indicates that 90% of mothers' emotional reactions have to do with concern for their child's well-being, followed by a preoccupation with the effects the abuse may have on herself, as well as feeling angry towards the abused child for the situation's occurring. There is an obvious link between mothers' actions and their emotions. For example, the more concern the mother has for the child, the more protective action taken for the child (Gomez-Schwartz, Horowitz & Cardarelli, 1990). Actions also influenced the reactions of the abused child and other family members. For example, a mother who believed her child's abuse disclosure and took action to protect the child from the perpetrator may have built confidence in the victim and maintained an open channel of communication between mother and child.

Other family members may have also worked to protect the child, while being more likely to have communicated their thoughts and feelings about the abuse. If a non-supportive action was taken, the sexual abuse may have continued and the family may have begun or continued to treat the abuse as a family secret.

Culture also plays a critical role in the non-offending parents and other family members reactions to both intra-familial and extra-familial sexual abuse. Research conducted by Ramona Alaggia (2001) asserted that cultural factors played a significant role in how mothers understood the sexual abuse of their child, as well as influencing the mothers' supportive or less supportive actions following the sexual abuse disclosure. Cultural and religious concepts concerning issues of forgiveness, cultural beliefs about preserving the family, and value conflicts between mothers and service providers

Conclusion

Disclosure of child sexual abuse is a highly complex and an unending process that for many never ends. Non-disclosure or delayed disclosures pose a significant risk for children and families and present a challenge for professionals. When children do not disclose or delay disclosure, there is a possibility of continued abuse and this might provide little or no possibility for intervention. Attitude and perception of parents and caregivers to disclosure of abuse has impact on mental health of abuse victims.

References

Ahrens, C., Campbell, R., Ternier-Thames, N., Wasco, S. & Sefl, T. (2007). Deciding whom to tell: Expectations and outcomes of rape survivors' first disclosures. *Psychology of* Women *Quarterly*, 31(1), 38-49. doi:10.1111/j.1471-6402.2007.00329.x.

Alade, A. O., (2015) Dialectical behaviour and cognitive processing therapies in the reduction of emotional stress among sexually abused female in-school adolescents in Ibadan metropolis. Unpublished PhD Thesis, University of Ibadan. Ibadan. Nigeria.

Alaggia, R. & Kirshenbaum, S. (2005). Speaking the unspeakable: Exploring the impact of family dynamics on child sexual abuse disclosures. *Families in Society, 86*, 227-234.

Arata, C. M. (1998). To tell or not to tell: current functioning of child sexual abuse survivors who disclosed their victimization. Child Maltreatment, 3, 63–71.

Bandura, A. (1986). Social foundation of thought and action: a social cognitive theory. Englewood Cliffs, NJ: Prentice-Hall.

Bandura, A. (1989). Social cognitive theory. In: R. Vasta (Ed.), Annals of child development: six theories of child development (vol. 6, pp. 1–60). Greenwich, CT: JAI.

Banyard, V. L., Arnold, S. & Smith, J. (2000). Childhood sexual abuse and dating experiences of undergraduate women. *Child Maltreatment, 5*(1), 39-48.

Banyard, V., Moynihan, M., Walsh, W., Cohn, E. & Ward, S. (2010). Friends of survivors: The community impact of unwanted sexual experiences. *Journal of Interpersonal Violence*, 25(2), 242-256. doi:10.1177/ 0886260509334407.

Banyard, V., Williams, L. M. & Siegal, J. A., (2001). The long-term consequences of child sexual abuse: An exploratory study of the impact of multiple traumas in a sample of women. Journal of Traumatic Stress, 14, 607–715.

Barter, C. (2009). In the name of love: Partner abuse and violence in teenage relationships. *British Journal of Social Work*, 39(2), 211 - 233.doi:10. 1093/bjsw/bcm127.

Barth, J., Bermetz, L., Heim, E., Trelle, S. & Tonia, T. (2013). The current prevalence of child sexual abuse worldwide: a systematic review and meta-analysis. *International Journal of Public Health, 58*(3), 469-483.

Blau, P. M. (1964). Exchange and power in social life. New York: Wiley.

Bolan & Lamb, (2004).

Bolen, R. & Lamb, J. L. (2007). Can non offending mothers of sexually abused children be both ambivalent and supportive? *Child Maltreatment, 12*(2), 191-197.

Browne, A. & Finkelhor, D. (1986). Impact of child sexual abuse: A review of the research. *Psychological bulletin, 99*(1), 66-77.

Byron, T. (2010). Do we have safer children in a digital world? A review of progress since the 2008 Byron review. DCSF-00290.

Campis, L. B., Hebden-Curtis, J. & Demaso, D. R. (1993). Developmental differences in detection and disclosure of sexual abuse. *Journal of the American Academy of Child and Adolescent Psychiatry,* 32, 920–924.

CEOP (Child Exploitation and Online Protection). (2012). A Picture of Abuse. A thematic assessment of the risk posed by those who possess indecent images of children. Executive Summary. 1–15. Available from: http://www.ceop.police.uk/Documents/ceopdocs/ CEOPIIOCTA Executive Summary. pdf [last accessed 12 January 2013].

Collings, S., Griffiths, S. & Kumalo, M. (2005). Patterns of disclosure in child sexual abuse. *South African Journal of Psychology, 35*(2), 270-285.

Cutajar, M. C., Mullen, P. E., Ogloff, J. R. P., Thomas, S. D., Wells, D. L. & Spataro, J. (2010). Psychopathology in a large cohort of sexually abused children followed up to 43 years. Child Abuse and Neglect, 34, 813–822.

Daignault, I. & Hébert, M. (2009). Profiles of school adaptation: Social, behavioral and academic functioning in sexually abused girls. *Child Abuse & Neglect*, 33(2), 102-115. doi:10.1016/j.chiabu.2008.06.001.

Filipas, H. H. & Ullman, S. E. (2006). Child sexual abuse, coping responses, self-blame, posttraumatic stress disorder, and adult sexual revictimization. *Journal of Interpersonal Violence, 21*, 652-672.

Finkelhor, D. Shattuck, A., Turner, H & Hamby, S. (2014). The Lifetime Prevalence of Child Sexual Abuse and Sexual Assault Assessed in Late Adolescence. *Journal of Adolescent Health Article in press xxx (2015)* 1-5.

Finkelhor, D., Hotaling, G., Lewis, I. & Smith, C. (1990). Sexual abuse in a national survey of adult men and women: Prevalence, characteristics, and risk factors. Child Abuse and Neglect, 14, 14–28.

Frese, B., Moya, M., Megias, J. L. (2004). Social perception of rape: How rape myth acceptance modulates the influence of situational factors. *Journal of Interpersonal Violence,* 19, 143- 161.

Ghetti, S. & Goodman, G. S. (2001). Resisting distortion. *Psychologist, 14,* 592–595.

Goodman-Brown, T., Edelstein, R., Goodman, G, Jones, D. & Gordon, D. (2003) Why children tell: A model of children's disclosure of sexual abuse. *Child Abuse & Neglect.* 27: 525- 540.

Hebert et al., 2007).

Hebert, M., Daigneault, I., Collin-Vezina, D. & Cyr, M. (2007). Factors Linked to Distress in Mothers of Children Disclosing Sexual Abuse. *Journal of Nervous and Mental Disease, 195*(10), 805-811.

Hershkowitz, I., Lanes, O. & Lamb, M. E. (2007). Exploring the disclosure of child sexual abuse with alleged victims and their parents. *Child Abuse & Neglect, 31*, 111-123.

Hillenbrand-Gunn, T., Heppner, M., Mauch, P. & Park, H. (2010). Men as Allies: The efficacy of a high school rape prevention intervention. *Journal of Counseling Development*, 88(1), 43-51. Retrieved from PsycINFO database.

Jensen, T., Gulbrandsen, W., Mossige, S. Reichelt, S. & Tjersland, O. A. (2005) Reporting possible sexual abuse: A qualitative study on children's perspectives and the context for disclosure. *Child Abuse and Neglect* 29(12):1395-1413.

Jones, D. (2000). Editorial: Disclosure of Child Sexual Abuse. *Child Abuse & Neglect 24*: 269- 271.

Kellogg, N. D. & Huston, R. L. (1995). Unwanted sexual experiences in adolescents: Patterns of disclosure. *Clinical Pediatrics, 34,* 306–312.

La Rooy, D. J. Malloy, L. C. & Lamb, M. E. (2011). The development of memory in childhood. In M. E. Lamb, D. J. La Rooy, L. C. Malloy & C. Katz (Eds.), *Children's Testimony: A Handbook of Psychological Research and Forensic Practice* (pp. 49-68). Wiley- Blackwell.

Lamb, M. E., Malloy, L. C. & La Rooy, D. J. (2011). Setting realistic expectations: Developmental characteristics, capacities, and limitations. In M. E. Lamb, D. J. La Rooy, L. C. Malloy & C. Katz (Eds.), *Children's Testimony: A Handbook of Psychological Research and Forensic Practice* (pp. 15-48). Wiley-Blackwell.

Lamb, M. E., Sternberg, K. J. & Esplin, P. W., (2000). Effects of age and delay on the amount of information provided by alleged sex abuse victims in investigative interviews. *Child Development, 71*, 1586–1596.

Lamb, M. Orbach, Y., Hershkowitz, I., Horowitz, Abbott, C. (2007) Does the type of prompt affect the accuracy of information provided by alleged victims of abuse in forensic interviews? *Applied Cognitive Psychology* 21(9):117-130.

Lamb, M. E. & Garretson, M. E. (2003). The effects of interviewer gender and child gender on the informativeness of alleged child sexual abuse victims in forensic interviews. *Law and Human Behavior, 27*, 151-171.

Livingston, J., Hequembourg, A., Testa, M. & VanZile-Tamsen, C. (2007). Unique aspects of adolescent sexual victimization experiences. *Psychology of Women Quarterly*, 31(4), 331-343. doi:10.1111/j.1471-6402.2007.00383.x.

Livingstone, S., Haddon, L., Gorzig, A. & Olafsson, K. (2010). Risks and safety for children on the internet: The UK report. Full Findings from the EU Kids Online Survey of UK 9–16 Year Olds and their Parents. Available from: http:// www.eukidsonline.net [last accessed 12 January 2013].

London, K., Bruck, N., Wright, D., Ceci, S. (2008) Review of the Contemporary Literature on how children report sexual abuser to others: Findings methodological issues, and implications for forensic interviewers. *Memory,* 16(1): 29-47. Article in press doi:10:1002/car.2280 (2013)

London, K., Bruck. M, Ceci., Shuman, D. (2005). Disclosure of Child Sexual Abuse: What Does the Research Tell Us About the Ways That Children Tell? *Psychology, Public Policy, and Law 11*(1): 194-226.

Lovett, B. B. (2004). Child Sexual Abuse Disclosure: Maternal Response and other Variables Impacting the Victim. *Child & Adolescent Social Work Journal 21*(4): 355-371.

Martin, E., Silverstone, P. (2014). How Much Child Sexual Abuse is "Below the Surface," and Can We Help Adults Identify it Early? *Frontiers in Psychiatry 4*: 58-58.

McElvaney. R. (2002) Delays in reporting childhood sexual abuse and implications for legal proceedings. In sex and Violence " the Psychology of Crime and Risk assessment, Farrington, Dp, Hollin, CR, McNurran M(eds) Routledge, London: 138-153.

Mian, M., Wehrspann, W., Klajner-Diamond, H., Labaron, D. & Winder, C. (1986). Review of 125 children 6 years of age and under who were sexually abused. Child Abuse and Neglect, 4, 223–229.

Mullen, P. E., Martin, J. L., Anderson, J. C., Romans, S. E. & Herbison, G. P. (1993). Childhood sexual abuse and mental health in adult life. *British Journal of Psychiatry, 163,* 721-32.

Mullens, P. E., Martin, J. L., Anderson, J. C., Romans, S. E. & Herbison, G. P. (1996). The long- term impact of the physical, emotional and sexual abuse of children: A community study. Child Abuse and Neglect, 20, 7–21.

Orbach, Y. & Lamb, M. E. (2007). Young children's references to temporal attributes of allegedly experienced events in the course of forensic interviews. *Child Development, 78*(4), 1100-1120. 117.

Orbach, Y., Hershkowitz, I., Lamb, M. E., Sternberg, K. J., Esplin, P. W. & Horowitz, D. (2000). Assessing the value of structured protocols for forensic interviews of alleged child abuse victims. *Child Abuse & Neglect*, *24*, 733-752.

Orbach, Y., Shiloach, H. & Lamb, M. E. (2007). Reluctant disclosers of child sexual abuse. In M.-E. Pipe, M. E. Lamb, Y. Orbach & A.-C. Cederborg (Eds.), *Child Sexual Abuse: Disclosure, Delay, and Denial* (pp. 115-134). Mahwah, NJ: Erlbaum.

Paine, M. L. & Hansen, D. J. (2002). Factors influencing children to self-disclose sexual abuse. *Clinical Psychology Review, 22,* 271–295.

Pipe, M. E., Lamb, M. E., Orbach, Y., Sternberg, K. J., Stewart, H. & Esplin, P. W. (2007). Factors associated with nondisclosure of suspected abuse during forensic interviews. In M. E. Pipe, M. E. Lamb, Y. Orbach & A. C. Cederborg (Eds.), *Child sexual abuse: Disclosure, delay and denial* (p. 77-96). Mahwah, NJ: Lawrence Erlbaum Associates Inc.

Pipe, M.-E., Lamb, M. E., Orbach, Y. & Cederborg, A.-C. (2007). *Child Sexual Abuse: Disclosure, Delay, and Denial*. Mahwah, NJ: Erlbaum.

Priebe, G. & Svedin, C. (2008). Child sexual abuse is largely hidden from the adult society: An epidemiological study of adolescents' disclosures. *Child Abuse & Neglect 32*(12): 1095- 1108.

Putnam, F. W. (2003). Ten-year research updates review: Child sexual abuse. *Journal of the American Academy of Child & Adolescent Psychiatry*, *42*(3), 269-278.

Roesler, T. (1994). Reactions to disclosure of childhood sexual abuse: the effect on adult symptoms. *The Journal of Nervous and Mental Disease* (182): 618-624.

Romano, E. & De Luca, R. V. (2001). Male sexual abuse: A review of effects, abuse characteristics, and links with later psychological functioning. *Aggression and Violent Behaviour*, *6*, 55-78.

Royal College of Psychiatrists. (2012). Child abuse and neglect –The emotional effects: Information for parents, carers and anyone who cares for young people. Mental health and growing up factsheet. Royal College of Psychiatrists. March. Available from: http://www.rcpsych.ac.uk/ expertadvice/youthinfo/parentscares/parenting/childabuseandneglect.aspx [last accessed 12 January 2013].

Sauzier, M. (1989). Discloure of child sexual abuse: For better or for worse. Psychiatric Clinics of North America. 12:455-469.

Shackel, R. (2009). Understanding Children's Medium for Disclosing Sexual Abuse: A Tool for Overcoming Potential Misconceptions in the Courtroom. *Psychiatry, Psychology and Law,* 16(3): 379-393.

Smith, D., Letourneau, E., Saunders, E., Kilpatrick, D., Resnick, H., and Best, C. (2000). Delay in disclosure of childhood rape: results from a national survey. *Child Abuse & Neglect 24* (2): 273-287.

Sorenson, T., and Snow, B. (1991). The process of disclosure in child sexual abuse." *Child Welfare 70*: 3-15.

Summit, R. (1983) The child sexual abuse accommodation syndrome. *Child Abuse and Neglect* 7(2):177-193.

Summit, R. (1992). Abuse of the child sexual abuse accommodation syndrome. *Child Abuse & Neglect*, 24:689-700.

Ullman S. (1996). Social reactions, coping strategies, and self-blame attributions in adjustment to sexual assault. *Psychology of Women Quarterly*, *20*, 505-526.

Ullman, S. (2003) Social Reactions to Child Sexual Abuse Disclosures: A critical Review. *Journal of Child Sexual Abuse* 12(1)89-121.

Ullman, S. & Filipas, H. (2005) Gender differences in social reactions to abuse disclosures, post- abuse coping, and PTSD of child sexual abuse survivors. *Child Abuse & Neglect* 29 (2005) 767–782.

In: Caregivers
Editor: Adrienne Lloyd
ISBN: 978-1-63483-909-9

Chapter 6

REFLECTING ON A DECADE OF RESEARCH WITH CAREGIVERS OF CHILDREN IN HIV-AFFECTED SOUTHERN AFRICAN COMMUNITIES: A STORY OF HARDSHIP, RESILIENCE AND HOPE

Marisa Casale**, PhD
Senior Researcher, Health Economics and HIV/AIDS Research Division (HEARD), University of KwaZulu-Natal, South Africa

ABSTRACT

This chapter recounts the author's experiences and discusses empirical findings deriving from her research work with caregivers of children, since 2006, in HIV-affected Southern African communities. The author's entry into these caregivers' world commenced with multi-country qualitative research in South Africa and Malawi, aimed at better understanding and defining vulnerability in Southern Africa. What she observed and learned through her contact with households and communities would lead her to spend over five years conducting mixed methods research to explore the potential protective role of (family and community) social support for caregiver and child health. This chapter aims to combine the scientific with the experiential, to tell a story of challenges and resilience, despair and hope: a story that unravels over time through insights provided by both anecdotal and empirical information, as well as the author's own observations, questions and reflections. It concludes with suggested foci for future health and social support research and interventions with caregivers and children in Southern Africa.

INTRODUCTION

Since 2006, through my work at the Health Economics and HIV/AIDS Research Division (HEARD) at the University of KwaZulu-Natal (UKZN), I have been conducting research

* e-mail: Marisa.Casale@vodamail.co.za.

with caregivers of children in Southern Africa, mainly in South Africa's KwaZulu-Natal province. This province, my province of birth, is one of the areas of South Africa, and the world, that has been most affected by the HIV epidemic.

This research work has taken me, my colleagues and our project teams to some of the most resource-deprived informal urban and rural settlements in the province, where caregivers and their families wake up every day to deal with many challenges that many of us would find overwhelming in isolation – stresses such as income poverty, poor shelter, food insecurity, HIV and other illness, abuse and violence.

My entry into these caregivers' world commenced with multi-country qualitative research in South Africa and Malawi, aimed at better understanding and defining vulnerability in Southern Africa, and eventually led me to spend over five years conducting mixed methods research in order to explore the potential protective role of (family and community) social support for caregiver and child health.

The purpose of this chapter is to recount and reflect on this journey, by discussing my experiences and the empirical findings deriving from my research work over the past decade. This chapter therefore aims to combine the scientific with the experiential, to tell a story of challenges and resilience, despair and hope: a story that unravels over time through insights provided by both anecdotal and empirical information, as well as my own observations, questions and reflections. I conclude by highlighting areas and issues that I feel are important for future caregiver and child health research and interventions in Southern Africa.

A Decade of Research with Caregivers of Children in HIV-Endemic Southern Africa

Inspired by the Strength and Resourcefulness of Caregivers

I always knew that I wanted to work in my home country, inspired by the idea of using my skills to somehow contribute to poverty alleviationand human development. I hadn't planned to do this through research though, and the 2005 job opportunity in a health research unit in my home city had taken even me by surprise. My previous professional experience was in development finance and banking, and I had a broad interest in human development, but certainly not specialist knowledge in health. So when, in late 2005, I contemplated the prospect of spending the next few years of my life working in poor, HIV-affected households, I wondered whether I would be up to this challenge, technically and emotionally. I had been away from my home country for about thirteen years, mainly in Europe, and although I had spent some time working in microfinance in remote rural communities in South America, this was hardly comparable to the situation I knew awaited me in my own province. I knew I would be confronted with households where there would be many orphaned and ill children, mourning of deceased family members, sick or dying adults, and individuals left behind with the overwhelming responsibilities of caring for children and the ill, tying up debts and affairs of the deceased and supporting the household through whatever forms of available income.

Understandably, I imagined finding despair and suffering, and expected to be left with a sense of grief and distress myself, which I had accepted as a necessary consequence of this work. Yet to my surprise this was not (at least entirely) the case. Despite the hardship and distress I witnessed, each time we drove off from a township or rural informal settlement, I was filled with an increasing sense of determination, admiration for the people I had encountered, optimism and perhaps even a newfound belief in humankind. This, despite the undeniable hardship encountered and the fact that the logistics of conducting field research in – especially more remote – communities were admittedly far from easy, and we (I and the broader research teams) had on many an occasion found ourselves having to manage unforeseen challenges and emergencies. [1].

What provoked these feelings of respect and optimism was my interaction with caregivers – in many cases grandparents or even great-grandparents – and their children. I found myself interviewing older caregivers, mainly women, who were 'ordinary' individuals doing the extraordinary, by any society's standards: for example, women in their late 40s, 50s, 60s, but even 70s, 80s and 90s, looking after their households, tending a garden in the backyard to grow their own vegetables, simultaneously caring for a large number of foster children, and in some cases still partaking in income-generating work to sustain their extended family's livelihood.

Of course, the challenges they were facing, including risks to their own often compromised health, were evident. But, in most cases, these caregivers did not express their experiences as a desperate situation, or merely dwell on their hard luck in life. Rather, their presentation of the hardship faced was almost always tempered with positive experiences and qualities. These included resilience, warmth, an appreciation for the positive dimensions of their situation (including the opportunity to care for children and joy they derived from these activities), and a fiery determination to do their best to sustain their households and see their children established before they passed away.

This led me to develop and want to communicate a more nuanced perspective of the experience of caregiving in HIV-endemic resource-deprived contexts. For example, in a 2011 article published in the *Ageing and Society* journal, I argued that those of us contributing to the development of evidence on caregiving and HIV needed to seek to provide more nuanced analyses that reflected not only the adverse effects of HIV and caregiving, but also the positive responses, perspectives and experiences of caregivers that (co)existed with these (M Casale, 2011).

My focus in this particular article was older caregivers, and I wanted to challenge the stereotype of older carers or 'rural African grandmothers' as passive victims of a changing world, rather than key agents of change. To more effectively convey these messages and provide a human dimension to the 'issues' emerging from qualitative work, conducted over 2006-2007 with caregivers of children living in HIV-endemic semi-rural Northern KwaZulu-Natal[2], I decided to include the narratives of two female participants, constructed from four

[1] These challenges included difficult buy-in processes among tribal and government authorities, hostility towards the research team (in extreme cases being accused of being Satanists and chased out of research communities), being held hostage in classrooms, and spending many hours under the scorching sun lost on sand paths while looking for the nearest rural homesteads. These experiences are beyond the scope of this chapter but we felt significant enough to document and share with the broader research community, so they have been described in detail in previous publications (M Casale, Flicker, & Nixon, 2011; M Casale, Lane, Sello, Kuo, & Cluver, 2013).

[2] This qualitative research was conducted in the Amajuba district of Northern KwaZulu-Natal and was part of a larger study. The broader study was a collaborative effort between the International Food Policy Research Institute (IFPRI), the University of Cape Town, the Health Economics and HIV/AIDS Research Division (HEARD) at the University of KwaZulu-Natal and the Institute for Policy Research and Social Empowerment (IPRSE) in Malawi. It feeds into a body of ongoing research designed to improve knowledge of, and responses

in-depth interviews over a period of six months. These stories were then related to the findings of the broader study and the existing literature on caregiving, resilience and HIV. They highlighted both the strength and resourcefulness of (mainly older) caregivers in responding to adversity to ensure their families' survival and their leadership role in affronting HIV and related stigma within their own families.

Take for example, the story of Zandile[3], a 48-year old carer living in a semi-urban area in Northern KwaZulu-Natal and looking after four grandchildren and one biological child. After losing both her daughters to AIDS, Zandile had to leave her job as a domestic worker to take care of their children. She was forced to use savings from her previous work to pay for the funerals and initially for food for the household. In order to support her family, Zandile started running a tuckshop, growing and selling her own vegetables and using the child grants and disability grant received[4] (as a result of a health condition, which she describes as acute, debilitating bodily pains that last for up to ten days at a time). She deposited whatever (little) money she was able to put aside in savings accounts opened for her children's education. She described her greatest hope as that of seeing her children married and with jobs before she died 'to see and be proud of raising them.' Her more immediate wishes were to be able to buy her children items such as a basket-ball pole or computer.

Zandile's story clearly demonstrated how older carers were ensuring their families' survival through their strength and resourcefulness, and taking pride in their roles as 'surrogate' parents - despite the significant material and emotional stresses they were facing. Zandile's main concerns and hopes were centred around her children's immediate and longer-term happiness and security – which would accentuate her sense of fulfilment deriving from her role as surrogate mother.

Like Zandile, many other caregivers I interviewed were diversifying sources of income and strategies for coping; these included running small shops, growing vegetables for household consumption and sale, accessing and stretching grants, negotiating payment of school fees through instalments, selling 'muti' or traditional medicines and belonging to a 'food stokvel' (informal support group that purchases food in bulk and provides loans to members to purchase food). I will never forget one feisty grandmother, carer of 13 children, who proudly told of how she was still working at the age of 90, cleaning people's yards, to supplement the pension she received. She argued that there were a lot of employment opportunities available but that many young people were simply not hard-working enough. Thinking of my own grandmother, who at the time was nearing 90, still self-sufficient and energetic for her age, I could not imagine her having to take on income-generating work and

---

to, deteriorating livelihood conditions in sub-Saharan African populations. For further reading on the methodology and findings of this study: (M Casale, Drimie, Quinlan, & Ziervogel, 2009).

[3] Participants were given pseudonyms to ensure anonymity.

[4] Social grants are a key component of the South African government's social security system, which has the developmental objectives of reducing poverty amongst vulnerable and low-income groups and increasing investment in health, education and nutrition (Samson et al., 2004). There are different types of social security grants in South Africa, for example: the State Old Age Pension, the Disability Grant (for adults living with disabilities) and grants received for children, including the Child Support Grant (paid to primary caregivers of children to provide for basic needs) and the Foster Child Grant (paid to caregivers who have taken in foster children). Eligibility criteria for all of these grants take into account household financial status, and there are set maximum asset and income thresholds. This system is widely recognised to be improving the welfare of recipients and studies document how these social grants reinforce developmental impacts within households and increase the likelihood of finding employment (Samson, et al., 2004).

care responsibilities for young adults, at a time when we needed to be focusing on caring for her and minimizing her pain and discomfort.

Thandi, another 46-year old study participant had quite a different story to tell, as she was caring for six of her own children. Two of her siblings were HIV positive but were responding to the disease in very different ways. Her brother was in denial, drinking a lot and refusing to be tested, although the family saw 'symptoms of HIV/AIDS' and he had lost his small child to AIDS five years earlier. Thandi explained that her brother was afraid of knowing his status and that 'he could kill himself' if he were to find out he was HIV-positive. Her sister had been falling ill frequently and had also refused to be tested; she was afraid of how she would be treated if her family and community found out about her status. Eventually Thandi's mother managed to convince her daughter to take an HIV test by going to get tested herself, and promising not to disclose her daughter's status to anyone (including other family members).

What struck me about Thandi's story was not the multiple cases of HIV in the same family, or the stigma experienced and feared – as these phenomena were sadly not unusual for households in her community – but, instead the way her mother had responded to it. For me, Thandi's story illustrated the decisive leadership role taken by a family elder in addressing HIV/AIDS within her own family, and in breaking the silence and confronting stigma. This was not an isolated case. Other older female carer participants in our study were addressing HIV prevention, treatment and stigma within their own families, for example by encouraging children or grandchildren to be tested, and breaking the silence to talk about the epidemic. This was counter-intuitive to me in some respects: I would have expected older, female members of these households to adopt a more 'conservative' approach and to be reluctant to engage with issues related to HIV and sex. In fact the literature shows that in many African communities (including isiZulu communities) referring to sex and to the HIV/AIDS epidemic could be considered a sign of disrespect (Harrison, Xaba, & Kunene, 2001; Leclerc - Madlala, 1999). Yet other researchers have argued that older persons have a key potential role as intermediaries in HIV prevention and treatment and interventions should take advantage of these 'assets' (Knodel, Watkins, & VanLandingham, 2002); older carers would also have a substantial interest in encouraging safe behaviour among their children and younger relatives and may also have the necessary "emotional and material leverage" (Knodel, et al., 2002). It should, of course, be noted that more than seven years have passed since we conducted this research. The situation in similar communities has undoubtedly changed considerably, with HIV becoming more and more normalised and less stigmatised; indeed there were already studies showing this trend around the time of this research (Ssengonzi, 2009). However, I believe the potential role of elders as 'intermediaries' and leaders in addressing discrimination and self-stigma remains under-valued.

Other aspects of caregiving, which emerged from this research work and are often overlooked, are the psychological and emotional 'rewards' of caring for children and the way in which these may contribute to a caregiver's resilience and emotional wellbeing. For example, our qualitative data included many testimonies of the pride, love and enjoyment derived from a carer role, despite the many difficulties encountered. Most caregivers spoke affectionately about the advantages of having the opportunity to live with and care for their children, the satisfaction they gained from doing things to please their children and the hopes they had for their children's future (M Casale, 2011). A 64-year-old grandmother, for example, explained: "We are like friends. We discuss matters. If one person is not around we miss each other. We pray together". Other research has also highlighted the importance of the caregiver-child bond, both in terms of the physical support provided by children, and the emotional bonds. It has been argued that caregiving roles can be deeply fulfilling; for example: perceived rewards from caregiving can buffer carer burnout; orphans can help carers cope with the loss of their deceased relatives; and children can support the family by "restoring reciprocal support networks" through their (future) labour and income (Demmer, 2006; Schatz, 2007). A review of qualitative research with HIV-positive mothers showed that, despite the increased burden of motherhood (including disclosure, child care and custody issues), being a mother also provided these women with support, self-esteem, and a reason to live and fight HIV infection (Gillespie, 2004).

My research and the broader literature prompted me to argue that "In order to support carers and their families at various levels … focusing not only on the challenges, but also on the positive qualities, experiences and perceptions of carers, can provide us with important spaces and opportunities for intervention. This should in no way seek to romanticise the vulnerabilities of this population nor ignore the longer-term risks of current 'coping', but rather aim to propose a more useful platform for interventions to take advantage of and build on… Evidence that African grandmothers are, in many cases, dynamic, resourceful women with agency and leadership qualities, able to respond to a modern world while continuing to embrace tradition, should be central in considering how and where to support them, as well as highlighting the importance of their active role and participation in such responses …" (M Casale, 2011, pp. 18-19). A similar argument was put forward by May Chazan, a Canadian researcher who had collaborated with HEARD in 2005-2006 and conducted similar qualitative research with caregivers who were also migrant traders at an urban inner city market in Durban. Chazan called for more nuanced and forward-looking analyses and interventions, that "recognise grandmothers as central to the society's thin safety net and that grapple with older women's complex and diverse vulnerabilities." In a 2008 paper, she argued that prevailing 'wisdoms' about grandmothers and AIDS in Southern Africa were not accurate and could obscure their struggles and vulnerabilities, but also strength and resilience that had buffered some of the negative consequences of HIV on children and society (Chazan, 2008).

The work of another author, Morten Skovdal, has, in recent years, put forward similar arguments around resilience and agency in HIV-affected communities, although from the perspective of children. He and co-authors have contended that HIV in Southern African communities has changed the roles and views of children, who are increasingly considered to be 'capable and competent' actors providing care and support to people living with HIV, and individuals who are central to the survival of households (Skovdal, Magutshwa-Zitha, Campbell, Nyamukapa, & Gregson, 2013). These children's agency and role in the community response to HIV therefore need to be recognised by interventions (Skovdal, et al., 2013), as opposed to simply representing them as victims of their circumstances at high risk for psychosocial health problems.

These considerations were partly what inspired the focus of the documentary film I would years later (2011-2012) have the opportunity to co-develop with colleagues, in a remote research site in Northern KwaZulu-Natal. The documentary, entitled "Manguzi:

Raising Children in Rural South Africa[5]," aimed to tell the 'untold' stories of men and women caring for biological and foster children in a deep rural community where antenatal HIV prevalence was almost 40% and life expectancy 43 years (Department of Health, 2008; Umhlabuyalingana Local Municipality, 2011). As part of a broader research study[6], this participatiory film explored caregivers' lived experiences: whether caring for orphaned children, or children infected with HIV, it exposed carers' experiences of overcoming great personal challenges, but also of strength and solidarity. The aim of working with multimedia linked to our research was to reach beyond academia to NGOS and development agencies, but also to a broader global audience including individuals facing similar challenges or wanting to know more about these caregivers' world. As indicated in the documentary, our survey research showed that 74% of households with children aged 10-17 in the area were caring for at least one orphaned child, highlighting how widespread the phenomena of orphaning and foster parenthood really were. Almost half of the caregivers reported some form of stigma or social exclusion, though a few indicated that people were becoming more knowledgeable and accepting with regard to HIV and TB. Caregivers spoke of the challenges and stigma related not only to HIV but also to disability and other health conditions. For example one carer with Albinism, who was both a father and grandfather, explained how lucky he considered himself since "a person who looks like me can live to have grandchildren." He explained that, a while back, Albino children were socially marginalised and in some cases even killed at birth in his community.

Despite the many difficulties they were facing, caregivers left the audience with messages of hope for the future – they spoke of the importance of solidarity from the community for children who needed care, of encouraging children to study and behave well, of not surrendering to illness as a permanently debilitating state, and of respecting each other and the land they lived on. An HIV-positive grandmother caring for five grandchildren, Dalimede, pleaded "if there is an orphan that comes running saying that he or she has no-one on earth, you must not say food is expensive or that you are poor and have no-one. Go and embrace that child. Stay with them because I stayed with them."

I found the strength and altruism embedded in these messages astounding. How could individuals who were ill and exhausted, whose own children went hungry on nights when there was no food or no-one well enough to cook, not be bitter towards the world, not be lamenting or asking for help from the State and external agencies – but instead envisaging the care of further children in need as (their) individual and community responsibility? While these positions were admirable, it was also clear that this situation was neither feasible nor sustainable. These individuals could not be left to take on further responsibilities, where they were battling to fulfil current child care needs and further compromising their own health. One of our final messages in the documentary film was: "Caregivers show enormous strength caring for children but also face many challenges. Communities, organisations providing services, government and all of us can support the wellbeing of these families." It was a

[5] Documentary film produced by Kuo, C, Casale, M and Naysmith, A in 2012. Entitled 'Manguzi: Raising Children in Rural South Africa.' This was funded and produced by the Health Economics and HIV and AIDS Research Division (HEARD), University of KwaZulu-Natal. It is freely available at the following link: https://www.youtube.com/watch?v=KnOAVf9iAY4.

[6] This refers to the 'Young Carers' study described in more detail further on. It consisted predominantly of survey research conducted in three South African provinces, to better understand the effects of familial HIV. See www.youngcarers.org.za.

simple – possibly banal – message, but an important one in a context where children and families were still going hungry, carers ploughed the fields despite their ill health and difficult climatic conditions, only a minority of people had formal work, and ill individuals still had to walk for kilometres on sand paths under a hot sun to reach a health facility, and possibly queue up for hours to see a nurse. Yes, many households were receiving social grants from the South African government – and this clearly put them in a better position than many families in other HIV-affected Southern African countries - but this was clearly not consistent enough or sufficient to meet their basic needs or those of the children in their care.

Multiple Stressors and Household Vulnerability

As explained above, my argument for greater attention paid to positive phenomena such as caregiver resilience and agency and the strength of the child-caregiver bonds was put forward with a view to better understanding and supporting them. In no way did I want to understate or disregard the enormous difficulties these (mainly female) carers faced on a daily basis, and the long term risks to themselves and their families. Never did I intend to convey the message that they were doing a great job and should be left alone to continue doing it. I hope that I did not unintentionally do so at any point.

Of course caregivers and their families faced many challenges, both physical and emotional. The more obvious ones were the consequences of poverty: inadequate shelter; food insecurity, worsened by erratic or extreme weather that destroyed subsistence crops. Beyond this, there were the less visible stressors. Study participants spoke about how their illnesses, the grief of having lost a child or young adult relative to HIV, and the stress and anxiety they experienced struggling to fulfil the financial and emotional needs of their children in severely resource-constrained conditions. In fact, carers' future hopes of seeing their children established (e.g., married or employed) before they died coexisted with the fear – especially amongst older carers – of not living to see this materialise; the concern that they would die before their (older) children were able to take care of themselves was an additional source of stress (M Casale, 2011). As explained by a 48-year-old grandmother: "My main concern is my children. If I die I don't know where they will go, since I'm the only one taking care of them."

Findings of research I was involved in, as well as other collaborative projects with children support by my research unit[7] and the broader literature on HIV and orphans and vulnerable children (OVC), continued to highlight the high burden of care on families in Southern Africa and the consequent risks for caregiver and child wellbeing. Most children in need of care were being absorbed by extended families; mainly women (Kuo & Operario, 2009) - and increasingly older adults, in the face of young adult mortality – were taking on the responsibilities of caring for children and the ill. On the one hand, it was argued that the extended family was a better option for children than institutions. These families were buffering some of the effects of HIV on children, allowing children to better manage risk, overcome suffering and move on after loss (The Joint Learning Initiative on Children and

[7] Earlier HEARD studies included the 'Joint Learning Initiative on Children and HIV/AIDS' (JLICA) and the 'Amajuba Child Health and Wellbeing research project' (ACHWRP). Further information and publications deriving from this work can be found on the HEARD website: www.heard.org.za.

HIV/AIDS, 2009). On the other hand, however, this situation was exerting a lot of pressure on caregivers and families' coping capacities, in a context of high HIV burdens and chronic poverty (The Joint Learning Initiative on Children and HIV/AIDS, 2009).

This was not surprising, unfortunately. Globally, a large body of literature shows that caring for multiple (biological and foster) children, in conditions of poverty and other livelihood stressors, is related to risks for poor caregiver physical and mental health. Research also suggests that the wellbeing of caregivers who are themselves living with HIV or other illness (Breuer, Myer, Struthers, & Joska, 2011), or caring for ill, foster and/or orphaned children may be particularly at risk. For example, a HEARD three-year longitudinal study with 600 orphaned and non-orphaned children in Kwazulu-Natal's Amajuba district[8] found that caregivers of orphaned children were more likely to care for a larger number of children, have poorer health, higher levels of chronic illness, more daily responsibilities and less adult support (George, Govender, Bachoo, Penning, & Quinlan, 2013). Through her doctoral survey work conducted in an urban township close to Durban, a visiting research associate, Caroline Kuo, showed worse mental health and general health and functioning for caregivers of orphaned (versus other) children (Kuo & Operario, 2011).

The extent of these mental health risks have sadly been confirmed by a number of empirical studies that have used psychometric validated scales to test for mental health conditions, such as anxiety or depression, among HIV-affected individuals in South Africa. Studies conducted with samples of HIV-positive or chronically ill adults, and/or with caregivers living in similar resource-deprived HIV-endemic communities, have found between 20% and 40% of these individuals to be experiencing mental health conditions (Hughes, Jelsma, Maclean, Darder, & Tinise, 2004; Kagee, 2008; Kuo & Operario, 2009). Through our Young Carers work, for example, we found that around 36% of the 2477 caregivers in our KwaZulu-Natal sample – mainly women - were at high risk of clinical depression and 49% anxiety. Our data show that the prevalence of these mental health conditions among HIV-positive caregivers was significantly higher than that of other ill caregivers, which was in turn higher than the prevalence among healthy caregivers. Given that even 'healthy caregivers' were living in an HIV-affected area and dealing with a number of stresses related to caregiving, health and difficult economic conditions (M Casale, Wild, Cluver, & Kuo, 2015), it is not surprising that these rates were well above the estimated average national prevalence rates for major depressive disorder (10%) and any mental health disorder (30%) in South Africa (Herman et al., 2009). There is also a strong gender element to these risks, as the majority of care responsibilities are borne by women. Our Young Carers KZN survey data in fact showed that rates of depression and anxiety were significantly higher for female caregivers than for males (for example, 39% males versus 51% females were experiencing anxiety (M Casale, Wild, Cluver, & Kuo, 2014)).

These findings are concerning not only for caregivers, but also for the children in their care, as poor caregiver mental and physical health has been shown to pose challenges for both parenting and child health (Stein, Ramchandani, & Murray, 2008). It was clear that, despite caregiver and family apparent resilience, the multiple stressors and burdens HIV-affected

[8] The 'Amajuba Child Health and Wellbeing research project' (ACHWRP) study ACHWRP was a collaborative effort between HEARD and the Center for International Health and Development (CIHD) at the Boston University School of Public Health (BUSPH). The overall objective of this research was to better understand the social and economic consequences of orphaning on school-age children (aged 9 – 15) in the Amajuba district.

households were increasingly having to deal with was leaving them more and more vulnerable to health, economic and (in the case of children) developmental risks. It was therefore important to better understand the nature of this vulnerability and how to strengthen these families.

This was in part the objective of the multi-country qualitative research I was involved in, through HEARD, over 2006- 2008 in Malawi and South Africa. This study, a collaboration with the International Food Policy Research Institute (IFPRI), was aimed at better understanding the concept of vulnerability in the context of HIV and multiple stressors in Southern Africa; one of the specific objectives was to determine whether caregivers were planning for their children's future (M Casale, et al., 2009). Using identical methodologies, we conducted multiple in-depth interviews with caregivers of children on three research sites: an urban marketplace and semi-urban township in South Africa, and a rural community in Malawi. After comparatively analysing our data as a team, we identified five phenomena that were strikingly common across the different research sites, which we referred to as 'symptoms' of vulnerability. These were: frequent bouts of minor illness among children; inability to make use of opportunities to deploy household labour (e.g., unemployment and inability to develop sufficient skills to fit requirements for employment); weakening of social networks (because of the difficulty of sustaining them or migration); food and nutrition insecurity; and the absence of long-term planning, including for the children's future (M Casale, et al., 2009). This study was qualitative and exploratory, so of course these 'symptoms' could not be generalised to broader populations or taken as indicators common to all Southern African communities. They did, however, contribute to the evidence aimed at directing further studies seeking to assess vulnerability in Southern Africa[9].

Part of the purpose of this work was to understand the strategies employed by caregivers and families to cope with stressors. Our data pointed to coping strategies such as reciprocity, diversification of income, but also marrying daughters off young and employing child labour (in the Malawian site) and selling household assets and livestock (M Casale, et al., 2009). Unfortunately some of these strategies, while providing short-term relief, risked negatively affecting households' longer-term human and financial capital, for example by compromising children's education or depleting savings and income-generating assets. This could in turn jeopardize the family's future resilience or ability to deal with crises that could arise in the future. Thus, we argued, a weakened ability to cope in the long run could lead to families being trapped in a vicious cycle of increasing vulnerability (Drimie & Casale, 2009). Of course this work directly and indirectly pointed to developmental risks for children. Their education and health would be compromised, but also the lack of parental planning and strained social networks, amidst an HIV epidemic and before the widespread availability of ART, raised the question of how the material and emotional needs of many children would be met in the not-too-distant future.

These findings, together with those of other empirical studies, contributed to the 'Joint Learning Initiative on Children and HIV/AIDS' (JLICA) work on Strengthening Families, on

[9] For example, the Southern African Vulnerability Initiative (SAVI) was comprised of scientists from various disciplines that worked together on a number of research projects since 2004 and represented a loose network. It included organizations such as the Stockholm Environment Institute (SEI), Clark University, the Health Economics and HIV/AIDS Research Division (HEARD) of the University of KwaZulu-Natal, Environmental and Geographical Sciences at the University of Cape Town and the International Food Policy Research Institute (IFPRI). See for example: (O'Brien, Quinlan, & Ziervogel, 2009).

which I collaborated through HEARD. The JLICA, a collaborative initiative between South African and international research institutions, engaged practitioners, policymakers, and scholars from around the globe in a multi-year collaboration focused on the needs of children affected by HIV/AIDS. Its work, consisting of problem-solving, research and analysis, was conducted by four interdisciplinary Learning Groups. Its final report, which pulled together findings of the various groups, was released in 2009 (The Joint Learning Initiative on Children and HIV/AIDS, 2009). While the JLICA report once again brought to light the central role that families and communities were playing in mediating the impacts of HIV on children and providing them with long-term assistance, it also showed how the long-run capacity of families to protect children could be fragile and uncertain (The Joint Learning Initiative on Children and HIV/AIDS, 2009). Studies highlighted the extraordinary burden that HIV, poverty and other social stresses were placing on families over time, and the risks of erosion of the extended family and community capacity to carry that burden (The Joint Learning Initiative on Children and HIV/AIDS, 2008). The JLICA report made recommendations for policy and practice, arguing that access to HIV services and support needed to be combined with a social protection agenda. And that children should be placed at the centre to spur development, by strengthening families, supporting community involvement and collaboration, and protecting the human capital of future generations (The Joint Learning Initiative on Children and HIV/AIDS, 2009).

Focus on Social Networks and Social Support for Health

Through my experiences in communities, over the period of 2006 – 2009, I observed the importance of reciprocity and social networks as household coping strategies, and listened to caregivers' concerns about how over-burdened these networks were becoming. In all three sites of our vulnerability study, respondents had reported strain within reciprocal relationships and told of how it had become increasingly difficult to find solace with friends and neighbours during food shortages, as everyone was experiencing similar difficulties (M Casale, et al., 2009). There were also indications of reduced capacity to participate in local means of mutual income support, such as stokvels and burial societies; many households simply did not have sufficient money to make the necessary regular contributions (M Casale, et al., 2009). This was particularly worrying, because of the importance of these types of associations for coping with crises, and the erosion of longstanding informal social security mechanisms.

I became more and more interested in better understanding the potential protective effects of (instrumental and emotional) support derived from these networks for the wellbeing of caregivers and their families. My particular interest in social relations and networks for health was partly a result of my personal experiences, specifically having had to deal with stressors during specific periods of my life, in the absence of a strong social network (e.g., because of having moved to a new country or area where I had not yet established social ties). Moreover, 'social capital' was a construct that had always interested me conceptually, since having read the work of authors such as Robert Putnam. Being of part Italian descent, I was intrigued by his investigation of social capital and civic involvement across Italian regions, and his conclusion that differences in social capital endowments could be explaining differences in economic development and democratic processes (Putnam, 1993). Putnam defined social capital as the "collective value of all 'social networks' and the inclinations that arise from these networks to do things for each other (Putnam, 2000)," and considered it central to building and maintaining democracy. Despite being a somewhat elusive meta-concept without a single agreed definition, social capital has attracted increasing interest among policymakers and practitioners, because of concerns around social marginalisation, and strong evidence of links between social interaction and wellbeing. In our environmental and vulnerability research, social capital was a central construct used to define one of the key livelihood capitals that households possessed (together with other assets, such as human, natural and financial capitals); these resources or capitals were understood to be closely linked to a household's coping capacity and resilience (M Casale, et al., 2009).

Going back to the situation of caregivers in Southern Africa, I was interested in how the functional nature of their social relationships and networks – the support provided – could have positive benefits for their wellbeing. 'Social support' is in fact a construct more frequently used in analyses conducted within disciplines such as sociology and psychology, to assess health benefits deriving from social networks. It is related, but slightly different to the concept of social capital. The positive role of social support in relation to health[10] has been defined as "… supportive relationships that directly provide something that people need to stay healthy or adapt to stress" (House, Umberson, & Landis, 1988, p. 302). This 'something' provided can embrace various types of support, such as emotional support (e.g., love and care), instrumental support (e.g., tangible items and practical assistance), affirmational or appraisal support (e.g., encouragement, being assured that one is doing a good job) and informational support (e.g., advice and information).

The strong potential role of social relations and support for health is undeniable, but recent evidence has shown it to be surprisingly strong. A meta-analysis conducted in 2010 showed social relations to be as important a determinant for health as well known, more tangible, risk factors, such as cigarettes or alcohol (Holt-Lanstad, Smith, & Layton, 2010). More broadly, there is a wealth of evidence showing a strong relationship between more received or perceived social support and better (mental and physical) health outcomes, among ill and healthy adults (House, et al., 1988; Sarason, Pierce, & Sarason, 1990; Thoits, 2011).

A consideration of the above literature, and my own experience in HIV-affected communities, led me to pose a number of questions: To what extent was the support and reciprocity caregivers received from their families, friends and communities protecting them and their households from further adverse consequences of HIV, poverty and other stressors? And what were the most important types of support or channels through which this was occurring? Who was providing this support and for how long could these strained reciprocal relations be sustained? Lastly, and importantly, what would happen to these caregivers and households if these networks were to fall away?

My growing interest in the importance of social networks and social support[11] for the health of HIV-affected caregivers and their households led me to dedicate about five years of

---

[10] It should be noted that social networks can also have negative effects on health and behavioural outcomes, including exclusion, negative peer pressure or influences and marginalisation. While I recognise this, my intention was to focus specifically on the support deriving from these relationships. Though less common, it is possible that even well-intended support may have negative unintended effects; this was not, however, an experience reported by caregivers who participated in my qualitative study (M Casale, 2013).

[11] Social support and social capital are not unrelated, but are slightly different dimensions and ways of conceptualising the functions and effects deriving from social networks and relations. Social capital is more commonly applied in economic research as it considered as a type of 'asset' that one can attempt to quantify;

my professional life as a researcher (2009 – 2014) to better understanding and documenting the potential protective effects of social support for caregiver health and wellbeing. My involvement in the Young Carers project[12] - a collaboration between the Health Economics and HIV/AIDS Research Division (HEARD), the South African government, NGOs and academic institutions such as Oxford and Brown universities - provided me with the opportunity to lead analyses which aimed to contribute to filling the knowledge gap on social relations and health in the Southern African region. The Young Carers South Africa research project was the world's first large-scale study of the impacts of familial HIV/AIDS on caregivers and children; this survey research, conducted in KwaZulu-Natal and another two South African provinces, aimed to identify risk and protective factors which could be directly targeted by government policy and programming in order to improve caregiver and child outcomes. I co-managed the survey research on the two (one urban and one rural) KwaZulu-Natal sites, through which I had the opportunity to collaborate with a diverse and dynamic international research team. Based on some of the questions I sought to address, indicated above, I designed the section of this survey that was dedicated to measuring the availability of (both instrumental and emotional) social support received by caregivers, and determining who their main support providers were. I subsequently developed and conducted a 'bolt-on' or ancillary qualitative study[13] with 24 purposively chosen[14] caregivers who had participated in the survey, to explain and further explore quantitative survey findings. More specifically, it aimed to explore perceived mechanisms and pathways explaining the protective effects of social support on health. We collected 2477 paired child-caregiver survey interviews across the two sites, and I conducted in-depth qualitative work with 24 caregivers. The combination of the quantitative and qualitative components made this the largest mixed methods study in the field of social relations and health conducted in Southern Africa.

A recent commentary publication in a special edition of the British Journal of Health Psychology (M Casale, 2015) pulled together and discussed the various interlinked findings from this body of work, most of which had previously been published through a number of separate articles. Both the quantitative and qualitative components of this work showed social support to play a protective role for mental health among this sample of caregivers – and pointed to possible indirect benefits on physical health (M Casale, et al., 2014, 2015; M Casale, Wild, & Kuo, 2013). Caregivers who reported having more social support were less likely to be experiencing symptomatic anxiety (M Casale, et al., 2014) and more likely to report better mental health (M Casale, Wild, Kuo, & Cluver, 2012, July-b). However, for some outcomes, findings showed differences between different groups of caregivers. For

social support is more commonly used in social sciences such as psychology and sociology, and usually refers to the amount and types of support provided and received through social networks.

[12] The project was a collaboration between HEARD, the universities of Oxford (UK) and Brown (US), various other South African universities, key South African national government departments and NGOs. Household survey research with caregivers and children was conducted in an urban and rural site in three South African provinces (6 sites altogether): KwaZulu-Natal, Mpumalanga and Western Cape. HEARD was a funder and research partner for the KwaZulu-Natal research component. Further information on the national project can be found at: www.youngcarers.co.za. Site selection criteria included a high HIV prevalence (ante-natal prevalence of over 30%) and a high score on the health and social deprivation index (Noble et al., 2006).

[13] This is the 'Social Support and Caregiver Health' study, funded by HEARD. Further information on this work and related outputs can be found on the HEARD project page: http://www.heard.org.za/research/social-support-and-caregiver-health.

[14] Sample selection criteria for the qualitative study were aimed at achieving a sample consisting of male and female caregivers, and HIV-positive and HIV-negative caregivers, who had participated in the survey research.

example, social support was significantly associated with a lower likelihood of depression specifically for female caregivers living with non-HIV related chronic illness such as diabetes, cancer and hypertension (M Casale, et al., 2015), but not for male caregivers or other female caregivers. This suggested that social support could also be buffering against effects of illness-related stressors on depression for female caregivers.

The qualitative study pointed to some of the processes or pathways that could be explaining the support and mentalhealth relationship found through the survey analysis. These processes included the perceived effects of support on psychological factors such as mastery and hope, and on coping strategies (M Casale, Wild, et al., 2013). For example, caregivers spoke of how the support they received gave them the courage to tackle difficult situations and hope for a better future. The qualitative findings also offered a few possible explanations for the protective effect of social support for depression among female caregivers with chronic illness: rumination – that is, repetitive thinking about the causes, consequences and symptoms of one's illness or other negative affect – was reported mainly by ill female caregivers, who also explained that social interaction (versus isolation), and being able to talk about their problems, helped them interrupt this negative cycle (M Casale, 2013). More broadly, rumination is considered a maladaptive form of coping that has been found to explain the relationship between more social support and less depression specifically among women (Butler & Nolen-Hoeksema, 1991). It is one of the phenomena that should be further explored, possibly by future survey research with similar populations. However, a question that the qualitative findings were not able to shed light on, is why the social support received did not appear to be buffering against depression among HIV-positive female caregivers, as it was for female caregivers with other chronic illness. It is possible that social factors, such as stigma, or physiological factors, such as neuropsychiatric conditions caused by effects on the central nervous system, could be hindering this potential role (M Casale, 2015; M Casale, et al., 2015; Mellins, Ehrhardt, Rapkin, & Havens, 2000). As such, it may be that the mental health effects of HIV were too strong for social support to have a sufficient effect (Mellins, et al., 2000). However, for now we do not have the answer – the above are simply hypotheses that would need to be tested.

The qualitative findings also indicated that caregivers perceived social support to be positively influencing their physical wellbeing. Caregivers perceived this to occur in various ways: as a result of the positive effects of social support on better mental health, by encouraging positive health behaviours (e.g., less 'bad' health behaviours such as smoking, drinking or unhealthy eating and greater treatment adherence) and by facilitating access to health facilities and services (e.g., lifts to health facilities, a friend or relative picking up medicine or looking after the children so that the caregiver could do so) (M Casale, Wild, et al., 2013). The survey analyses did not allow for conclusive findings on the potential effects of social support on physical health, mainly because of limited indicators of physical health. However, there would be scope for future research to test this relationship, and the potential pathways mentioned above.

Lastly, while not the key focus of this study, both the quantitative and qualitative findings spoke to the perceived importance of support providers with regard to health. The survey showed that caregivers were mainly receiving support from their partners, family members and friends or neighbours; however, a minority of caregivers reported other sources, such as church members and support groups, as their key sources of support. Here too there was a gender element. While men were receiving more support than women, women – especially wives, partners and other female relatives - were the ones providing most of the support to both male and female caregivers (M Casale, Wild, Kuo, & Cluver, 2012, July-a). While women were reporting more support from their families, men were receiving more support from their significant others (predominantly women) (M Casale, et al., 2012, July-a). This should be considered in light of the fact that women were also more commonly primary caregivers, both for children and the ill. They were therefore disproportionately taking on direct care activities and supporting other caregivers.

We then extended this work on social support and caregiver health further, to focus beyond effects on the caregiver, to potential effects of caregiver support on child health and wellbeing. This is an important phenomenon to understand, particularly for practitioners and policymakers dedicated to protecting child and family health in Southern Africa. However, very little work in this area has been conducted globally, and there are no known previous empirical studies investigating these relationships in the Southern African region. More broadly, our Young Carers survey findings reinforced the strong bonds that exist between caregiver and child wellbeing. For example, caregiver HIV-related activity limitation was shown to be linked to more care and housework tasks for children, lower school attendance and child hunger (L. Cluver, Kganakga, Kuo, & Casale, 2010). Poor parental supervision was found to be associated with higher levels of risk behaviour among children and adolescents (Kuo, Cluver, Casale, Lane, & Sello, 2011). Children caring for adult caregivers living with HIV were found to be at higher risk of contracting tuberculosis (L Cluver, Orkin, Moshabela, Kuo, & Boyes, 2013). Living in a family affected by HIV was shown to lead to worse child educational, sexual and behavioural outcomes, through pathways including factors such as parental disability, abuse, stigma, bullying and poverty (L. Cluver et al., 2013).

In the case of an analysis I led, we looked at whether there was a relationship between caregiver social support and adolescent psychosocial wellbeing. We measured adolescent adjustment, using adult caregiver reports to determine peer problems, hyperactivity, conduct problems, emotional symptoms and child prosocial behavior (M. Casale et al., 2015). Our findings showed how adolescents whose caregivers reported more social support were more likely to have better mental health and behaviour, especially more prosocial behaviour (i.e., voluntary behaviour aimed at helping or benefiting others[15]) and peer relationships (M. Casale, et al., 2015). These results have important broader implications for child health risk behaviours and educational and health outcomes, both during adolescence and later in life (M. Casale, et al., 2015). Difficulties with peers have, for example, been shown to place children at risk for school problems (Rubin, Bukowski, & Parker, 2006). Prosocial behaviour, instead, has been shown to be linked to academic success and positive peer relationships (Caprara, Barbaranelli, Pastorelli, Bandura, & Zimbardo, 2000) and fewer health-risk behaviors in adulthood (Carlo, Crockett, Wilkinson, & Beal, 2011; M. Casale, et al., 2015).

What was very surprising to me about these results was the strength of the relationships we found between caregiver social support and these child outcomes; these appeared to be considerably stronger than those found between caregiver social support and caregiver outcomes (i.e., caregiver mental health and parenting). In my mind, the links between caregiver social support and caregiver mental health were likely and almost expected. Yet to find even stronger associations for what I would have considered to be an indirect relationship

[15] This voluntary behaviour could include actions such as helping, sharing, donating, co-operating, and volunteering.

between caregiver support and *child* outcomes was a surprise to me. This suggested that caregiver social support was not influencing children's wellbeing solely or possibly even primarily through its effects on the caregiver's wellbeing and parenting, but through some other channel(s). This was reinforced by mediation analyses we conducted, which showed that a part of this relationship could indeed be explained through parenting, but that a good part of it could not (M. Casale, et al., 2015). We therefore had to consider other possible explanations as to why young adults in this sample whose caregivers received more tangible and emotional support from their informal support networks were experiencing less emotional and behavioural problems and showing more adaptive behaviour.

We argued that the availability of caregiver support could be, to some extent, an indicator of other dimensions of family dynamics and social relations, such as the dimension and quality of the caregiver or family support network, or the amount of adult support and positive interaction provided directly to the adolescent child by members of this network (M. Casale, et al., 2015). The caregiver or family support network could be influencing these adolescents through various potential mechanisms or channels. For example, 'co-parenting' or sharing of caregiving responsibilities among several adult and/or extended family members is not uncommon in similar communities. Adult friends or family members could be serving as role models to children and adolescents and they could be providing direct emotional support and guidance; moreover, interaction with a larger caregiver/family social network could be boosting adolescent psychological factors associated with resilience (e.g., self-efficacy), increasing socialization and a sense of connection to others; and leading to social monitoring and social control (M. Casale, et al., 2015; Eisenberg, Fabes, & Spinrad, 2006; Thoits, 2011).

In terms of implications for intervention research and practice, we argued that findings of this analysis both reinforced the importance of social support components within parenting interventions and pointed to scope for positive intervention on adolescent psychosocial wellbeing through the broader family social network. These findings and their implications are, in my mind, of particular relevance in developing world contexts such as HIV-endemic Southern African communities. Unfortunately, a large number of young children and adolescents in these communities have been affected, and continue to be affected, by parental death and caregiver illness and absence. The suggestion that there is considerable scope for influencing the psychological and social health of these children through interventions that go beyond the interaction between with their primary caregiver is a positive one, that can provide us with hope in the potential success of other channels through which to influence these outcomes (e.g., even in the case of orphaned children or 'young carers'). However, while we are increasingly aware of the links between child and caregiver wellbeing, we still have much to learn and understand about the links between child and caregiver support availability and support networks.

Although not the key focus of the qualitative study, a small amount of qualitative data did emerge to suggest possible pathways through which caregiver social support could be influencing child health. This data supported, to some extent, the survey findings described above. For example, caregivers perceived the social support they were receiving to positively affect their children's health and behaviour indirectly, by having a positive influence on their (caregivers') mental health, parenting and decision-making (M Casale & Crankshaw, In press). However, caregivers also spoke about direct interaction between key individuals in their social networks and their children. For instance, information, advice and encouragement provided by members of the caregiver's network, to caregivers and directly to children, were considered to have positive effects on both caregiver and child health (M Casale & Crankshaw, In press). Itshould be noted that these findings were based on participants' perceptions and on limited data, and would require further in-depth focused research to be better understood.

CONCLUSION: REFLECTION ON CAREGIVER NEEDS AND APPROACHES FOR EFFECTIVE INTERVENTIONS

What Do Caregivers Need?

It is clear that caregivers of biological, orphaned and other foster children in Southern Africa have been carrying out a very important and difficult role in the context of HIV, poverty, young adult mortality, and many other stressors. In doing so they have demonstrated extraordinary commitment and resilience. Many – older and/or foster caregivers – are raising a large number of children, and sacrificing their own time, resources and even health for their children's development. These carers and their families continue to attenuate the impact of HIV and other social stressors on children. But can we consider this a positive phenomenon or success? It is unfortunately also clear that their heroic efforts risk, with time, eroding their health, their material resources, their long-term ability to cope and possibly even the survival of their family. This will have adverse effects on the healthy development of the children in their care. As I have argued above, I believe we need to acknowledge the resilience, agency and successes of caregivers, to learn from and work with them to best intervene. But we cannot leave them alone to 'get on with it.' If we do not continue to protect and support them, and better support them, we will see the consequences of this for generations to come. It will be our failure as researchers, practitioners and policymakers. It is therefore without question that these caregivers need to be better supported. The question is how?

I certainly cannot claim to have an exhaustive answer to this question. But based on my experience and the findings of my work, I have some thoughts on caregiver support needs and factors that should be considered when planning to address these. What struck me from my experience on the ground is that at times what people need most are really the simplest things. Things that many of us take for granted, but are still missing or unattainable to many carers living in both urban and rural South Africa. And I have often reflected how many of these individuals' unmet needs likely haven't changed that much over the years, despite the seemingly ever-changing objectives and foci of global development agencies and funders.

I think back, for example, to a caregiver in Amajuba who had lost family members to HIV and whose own home had burned down in the past. She was clearly still traumatised and, concerned at her apparent distress at every interview, we asked her whether she would prefer to interrupt her participation in our study. She responded that having someone to talk to, who listened to her, who she knew would not stigmatise or share this sensitive information, was a release for her. She begged us to let her continue to participate. She simply needed someone who would listen, encourage and comfort her, without stigmatising.

I think back to a blind and diabetic older woman we interviewed in an urban township close to Durban. She felt abandoned by her own children who did nothing to help her. And since she could not access health facilities or fetch her medication on her own, or make herself proper food, she was left to sit in her home alone and slowly waste away. What she needed most was someone to accompany her to a clinic or hospital, fetch her medication for her and assist her in taking it correctly, and help her buy and prepare food. At the same time she would undoubtedly have needed emotional support. She spoke of how much better she felt after a phone call to her sister who lived in another city. She also needed someone to listen and talk to, to show care and provide her with encouragement and hope.

Yes, hope, a central but often under-estimated concept, especially to those of us primarily concerned with quantifiable aggregates or medical solutions. Yet in my qualitative research (M Casale, Wild, et al., 2013) – and other studies (Yadav, 2010) - hope emerged as one of the most important factors explaining the influence of informal (family and community) support on the health of HIV-affected individuals. As explained by a young mother with HIV living in an urban township near Durban "If you give them [HIV-positive individuals] hope, you have done everything, hope for them means 'I will survive'. It is very important because I can give you money, you can do whatever but if you tell yourself that 'I will survive', you will survive ... because when you are taking that pill, you are taking it because 'I want to get well'". This should not be at all surprising if we think about our own lives: the hope of things getting better, the vision of what we can achieve and become is often imperative in motivating us to struggle on or to act on many things. If we cannot 'see' the usefulness and potential consequences of our actions, we are unlikely to be motivated to take them. It always baffles me why, as scientists, we tend to forget this when trying to understand or influence the behaviour of others.

The needs I have described above refer mainly to emotional support and psychological wellbeing. Of course most of the caregivers I interacted with also faced significant material challenges, and could certainly do with further tangible support. However, it is important to recognise that South Africa has an extensive social grant system that – despite its limitations – has been central to supporting some of the most vulnerable households and, in particular - through child grants - households with children (Samson, et al., 2004). This distinguishes South African populations from many others on the continent, in that a large number of low-income households have the opportunity to access a social protection system that provides them with some level of subsistence income. There are, of course, households that fall into the 'gap' space, for example families with adults who are unemployed but too young to access pensions, unable to access disability or child grants for various reasons, and/or with too many children in their care for the child grants to make a substantial contribution to their livelihoods. Our research teams came across many of these households.

I think, for example, back to a grandmother caring for six children in an urban KZN township who told me, during an interview, that she did not know what she would give her children to eat the next day as they had run out of food. No-one in the household was employed and she had been to the priest to ask for assistance with food more than once. Although he had told her to come to him for help whenever she needed, she felt as though she could no longer burden him, as there were many other people in her parish in need.

These experiences of course raise ethical dilemmas for us researchers. We are not interventionists and cannot provide money or services, as much as we would like to help. All I could do in this case was offer the last packets of biscuits we carried as small tokens of our appreciation for participants' time. And of course report the case to social services in the hope that the household would be included among the list of families receiving food parcels, and then follow up with social services a few weeks later. But we knew from experience that often social services never did contact households, address their needs in time, or provide a solution in the long run – for whatever reason, whether under-resourced, inefficient or simply not committed enough. We knew that not everyone would be helped, that likely most wouldn't, and we also knew that despite reporting these cases there wasn't much we could do. What this and many other households needed most, in the short term, was to be linked to a food parcel programme and feeding schemes for the children. What they needed in the long run were sustainable grant and employment income.

How Can We Best Support Caregivers and Their Families? Suggestions for Effective Interventions

It is very difficult to provide generic indications for 'standard' effective health and psychosocial interventions for caregivers and/or HIV-affected populations, as there is no 'one-size-fits-all' solution. What works in any given context will depend on a number of factors, including the characteristics and needs of specific end-user populations, the available financial and social resources, and the outcomes targeted by the intervention. Of course, in order to determine whether an intervention is more or less effective one would need to evaluate it. Unfortunately, most evaluations of social support interventions for health carried out to date derive from the developed world, and these have, overall, shown mixed results (M Casale, 2013; Ertel, Glymour, & Berkman, 2010) – highlighting that indeed there is no simple solution.

There are also many different types of approaches and interventions aggregated under the umbrella term of 'social support interventions.' Most of these interventions include one or more of the following components: support groups or sessions; professional assistance (e.g., patient management, counselling, mentoring), education (including cognitive behavioural therapy); and measures intended to improve existing social relations or networks (see for example: Davies, Hortona, Williams, Martin, & Stewart, 2009; Mason & Vazquez, 2007; Szapocznik et al., 2004). Based on a review of social support interventions, Ertel et al. (2010) argue that, while there is some evidence of interventions improving networks and positive health behaviours through self-help groups and skills-building, many other initiatives have not provided evidence of long-term health benefits (Ertel, et al., 2010; Uchino, 2006). There may be a number of reasons for this, including the evaluation methodologies used, the limitations of the interventions themselves and the assumptions driving them. It has been argued, for example, these may not be affecting social support sufficiently, or intervening at the right time (Ertel, et al., 2010, p. 83). Moreover, some of these approaches may be quite resource intensive and likely not feasible for resource-deprived settings; examples include interventions designed to identify and influence social interactions between individuals and their social environment (Feaster et al., 2011; Szapocznik, et al., 2004).

Another important issue is that much of the empirical evidence on associations between social support, health and mortality – including my work - is based on longer term "naturally occurring social relationships" (Holt-Lanstad, et al., 2010) with individuals within a person's social network. Most social support interventions, instead, consist of support provided by health professionals or other people outside of the recipient's informal social network, and many are short-term (for example, a given number of sessions provided over a short period of time). A question that researchers and practitioners continue to struggle with is how to emulate and include aspects of naturally occurring social relationships in formal programmes (Holt-Lanstad, et al., 2010). This may be particularly relevant in the context of rural or semi-urban HIV-endemic Southern African communities for example, where difficult living conditions and socio-cultural norms often foster a strong sense of solidarity, communalism and social regulation (Gade, 2012; Mukorombindo & Coetzee, 2013). (Mukorombindo & Coetzee, 2013; Verhoef, 2001). However, based on the mixed experiences of success to date, it would seem that how best to achieve this remains the '100 dollar' question.

As indicated previously, I cannot claim to have the answers to these questions, and believe a lot more iterative applied and evaluation work will need to be done, in order for us to move closer to effective intervention solutions. However, I do have some reflections on the issues and approaches we should be considering moving forward, in planning to support caregivers and their families with health and support interventions. Below I discuss what I consider to be some of the key points, drawing from my own work and experience, and the broader empirical and evaluation literature on social support and health.

Review and Consider Approaches That Seem to Work (Better)

While there is no standard social support intervention that will be suitable in all contexts, it can be useful to look to the evaluation literature to identify approaches and components that have appeared to work – or at least to be more effective – in one or more settings. As indicated above, there is some evidence of positive outcomes of self-help and support groups. Reblin and Uchino (2008), for example, argue that support groups can be effective within health interventions because of the gaps they fill in supporting patient needs, and because of similar experiences shared by groups members (Reblin & Uchino, 2008); as a result, these groups can be sources of community, information and acceptance. The qualitative data from my social support research, described above, indicate that access to support groups (e.g., through clinics or other community channels) was perceived by caregivers to be an important source of instrumental, informational and emotional support, and to be having a positive effect on their mental health (M Casale, Wild, et al., 2013). These groups allowed them a safe space in which to share their concerns and experiences, be listened to, and to learn from others. Similarly, HIV-positive parents participating in intervention studies in the U.S. have also highlighted the health benefits of psycho-educational support groups, that combined self-care and caregiving information with longer-term informal interaction between individuals with similar stressors (Davies, et al., 2009; Mason & Vazquez, 2007).

Some interventions that impart psychosocial skills (e.g., that educate about disease and teach relevant social skills) have shown positive outcomes, such as decreased loneliness and social isolation, lower perceived impact of disease and better social integration (Reblin & Uchino, 2008). As indicated above, these may involve group support or sessions. However, several cognitive behavioural interventions through 'mentors' also show some promise. For example, a pilot peer mentoring programme and culturally adapted cognitive behaviour intervention (CBI), originally from the USA, showed positive effects on social support, coping and mental health among HIV-positive South African women; this programme was rolled out in conjunction with PMTCT in two South African townships, with the support of 'mentor mothers' (Futterman et al., 2010).

Lessons can also be drawn from the experience of interventions working with other types of caregivers, such as carers of the ill or the elderly, and broader adult populations. For example, a meta-analysis of interventions for family caregivers of older adults showed some positive effect for outcomes such as caregiver burden, depression, subjective wellbeing and ability, with psycho-educational and psychotherapeutic interventions showing the most consistent short term effects (Sorenson, Pinquart, & Duberstein, 2002). Intervention effects were, however, moderated by a number of factors, such as number of sessions, setting, age, gender and nature of the caregiver-recipient relationship (Sorenson, et al., 2002). Findings of a systematic review of support interventions targeting social isolation in older people indicate that the most effective interventions were those developed with a theoretical basis, those providing social activities or support through a group format, and those in which the beneficiaries of support were active participants (Dickens, Richards, Greaves, & Campbell, 2011); the authors conclude that future interventions addressing social isolation in similar populations should aim to incorporate these three elements. In developed world settings, case management through health facilities for vulnerable and ill populations have shown promise, by helping patients feel less socially isolated, providing emotional support and helping them navigate the medical and social systems (Davis, Tamayo, Fernandez, & Cresswell, 2012). Other studies have instead shown social skills training (focused on how to activate and improve social relations) to be effective in preventing depression, and improving mental health and strengthening social networks (Dalgard, Anstorp, Benum, & Sorensen, 1995; Kühner, 2003); however, once again, most of the evidence originates from high income countries.

Several recent social support initiatives have incorporated new technologies, such as online support fora or cellular text messaging. For example, a pilot study testing the effects of an internet-based intervention on low-income African American mothers showed promise in positively influencing parenting and health care utilization, by providing these mothers with a forum to share experiences and acquire information from nurses on caring for themselves and their children (Hudson, Campbell-Grossman, & Hertzog, 2012). Phone education and telephone support groups have also been found to increase quality of life and decrease depression among ill adults and older caregivers (Reblin & Uchino, 2008). It should, however, be noted that these types of interventions require access to the relevant technologies, as well as an ability and willingness to utilize them. Some may not be relevant or feasible in certain developing world contexts – particularly in poorer, badly serviced and/or more remote areas. At the same time, those interventions that are feasible could be particularly useful in cases where, for example, caregivers are geographically isolated or unable to move from their home to health facilities because of factors such as physical illness and disability, anxiety, caregiving responsibilities and limited transport options. Through my field research experience in rural communities in KwaZulu-Natal, I learnt that even in the most remote areas, where caregivers do not have accesses to electricity, running water or transport services, they almost always own or have access to a cellular phone.

In sum, there are a number of social support intervention evaluations that provide us with insight on approaches that have been successful or showed promise within or across populations. It is clear, however, that intervention research in this area still has a way to go and that programmes need to be further developed and refined and their longer-term benefits assessed. Also, as there is no 'one size fits all' solution, programmes that have been successful in high income countries may not necessarily be appropriate for very different contexts in the developing world, and would have to be adapted and assessed in these settings. Moreover, where interventions consist of multiple components, it is difficult to ascertain which of these components works or does not work (Reblin & Uchino, 2008). This understanding will require research explaining the contexts and mechanisms behind the relationship between social support and health (M Casale, 2015; Reblin & Uchino, 2008). We need to continue designing and implementing new interventions based on the needs of specific populations, obtaining feedback and evaluating them in order to refine them, and incorporating social support components into mainstream health interventions.

Lastly, interventions should not disregard potential gender differences. It has been shown that support networks, availability and sources can be different for men and for women, as can the effects of support. This was highlighted by our findings from the Young Carers survey research (for example showing the relationship between more social support and a lower likelihood of depression, specifically for women) and is reinforced by the broader literature (M Casale, et al., 2015; Kendler, Myers, & Prescott, 2005; Schraedley, Gotlib, & Hayward, 1999; Walen & Lachman, 2000; World Health Organisation, 2002). On the one hand, attention needs to be paid to the heightened burden of care and particular health risks and needs of female caregivers in resource-deprived communities, especially where they are disproportionately taking on familial caregiving responsibilities and providing support to other caregivers, while possibly receiving less support than their male counterparts (M Casale, et al., 2012, July-a). On the other, we need to take into consideration the potentially different types of support and mechanisms through which these may be generating health benefits for men and women.

Develop Multi-Faceted Interventions Containing Multiple Components and Types of Support

The evidence that is available on effective or promising social support initiatives for health, suggests that interventions consisting of multiple components and/or types of support are likely to be more effective. Previous studies indicate that health interventions working with caregivers, especially HIV-positive caregivers, should seek to combine both emotional and tangible support, for example: home-based care initiatives that provide advice, encouragement and comfort as well as practical assistance with health care, transport to health facilities and caregiving tasks (Davies, et al., 2009). This resonates with my own observations and the perspectives of caregivers who participated in my qualitative research. These carers spoke of the equal importance they would place on the various types of support received (e.g., emotional, instrumental, informational) and suggested that support interventions would be most effective where types of support were provided in conjunction (M Casale, Wild, et al., 2013). My findings suggest that, besides encouraging practical health behaviour and facilitating access to health resources, it would be important for health interventions to focus on strengthening resourcefulness factors, such as hope, and more active coping responses to stressors (M Casale, Wild, et al., 2013). They indicate that for HIV-positive caregivers in particular, positive encouragement and emotional support are central to increasing the likelihood of ART adherence. And that support interventions targeting HIV-positive, and especially female, caregivers should provide them with opportunities to socialize and talk about their experiences and concerns, to protect them from social isolation and the negative mental health effects of continuously thinking about their illness and imminent death (M Casale, Wild, et al., 2013). Companionship and someone to listen and talk to without being judged, have been found by other studies to be the types of support valued most by child-bearing mothers accessing formal health services (Taft & Brown, 2011). this suggests the need for a combination of 'non-professional' support with that offered by health workers.

Various other studies with caregivers of the ill or elderly have also pointed to a greater effectiveness of tailored and multi-component interventions (Acton & J., 2001; Gitlin et al., 2003; Lopez-Hartmann, Wens, Verhoeven, & Remmen, 2012; Reinhard, Given, N, & Bemis, 2008). For example, a systematic review of support services to relieve caregiver burden and improve mental health among informal caregivers of community-dwelling elderly, concluded that these caregivers were best supported through integrated support interventions, comprising elements such as respite care, group support and technology-based interventions (Lopez-Hartmann, et al., 2012). It was also argued that the content of the intervention needed to be adapted to the caregiver's physical, psychological and social needs, with the participation of the caregivers themselves (Lopez-Hartmann, et al., 2012). Other factors that have been associated with positive outcomes for family caregivers, to be included and assessed in future multi-component interventions, include care plans adapted to the caregiver's specific needs, knowledge and skill building, problem solving, counselling, appropriate referrals, and combinations of home-visiting and follow-up through channels such as the telephone or internet. Some of the desired outcomes would be to simultaneously boost caregivers' confidence and competency, reduce distress, assist them in navigating the health system and addressing care recipients' specific needs, and mobilizing supportive resources in their informal networks and formal services (Reinhard, et al., 2008).

Though not specific to social support, it is important to note that, more broadly, some of the most promising behavioural change and health intervention evaluations refer to multi-faceted programmes, combining livelihoods interventions with psycho-educational and behavioural components. For example, a study with poor women in rural Limpopo, South Africa, showed how a combined microfinance and participatory training intervention could lead to reductions in levels of intimate-partner violence (Pronyk et al., 2006), highlighting the potential of social and economic interventions to change risk environments (Pronyk, et al., 2006). Similarly, recent findings from a qualitative longitudinal cohort study of young men who participated in a gender transformative and livelihood strengthening intervention (the 'Stepping Stones and Creating Futures' intervention) showed perceived improvements in the men's livelihoods and relationships, suggesting a positive effect on gender dynamics despite a very difficult social environment (Gibbs, Jewkes, Sikweyiya, & Willan, 2015). The rationale behind these interventions is that in a developing world context of poverty and unequal gender power dynamics, economic empowerment is integral to increasing choices and agency, and reducing risks, particularly among women. Similarly, trying to positively influencing health outcomes of caregivers in poor households through emotional support, information and advice may be difficult and have limited effects if caregivers do not have the tangible resources to provide food and meet basic household needs, reach a health facility or pay someone else to look after their children while they access these services. Livelihood support – whether through grants, in-kind assistance or income-generating opportunities – may also be critical in certain circumstances.

In sum, there are many types of social support interventions that may combine multiple approaches or components. Perhaps the key question is which types of components to best include and combine in specific caregiver and HIV-affected populations. Attempting to address this question would require taking into account the specific characteristics, challenges and needs of the target population. It is noteworthy that many of the studies cited above refer to the usefulness of participatory interventions, that are locally designed and/or allow for the input of end-users. With reference to family caregivers, Reinhard et al. (2008), for example, argue that interventions must recognize professional or 'formal' caregivers and family caregivers as 'partners' in health care versus simply recipients, and engage them in care plans (Reinhard, et al., 2008).

Pay More Attention to the Child-Caregiver Relationship

When planning to intervene to support caregivers of children, the most obvious approach is to focus on the caregiver. However, it is also important to consider the child-carer relationship. At one level this means understanding how caregiver and child wellbeing are linked and influence each other. At another, this includes understanding how caregivers and children may be providing instrumental and emotional support to each other, and how their respective support networks and providers may be intertwined. These are important questions, particularly in many HIV-affected communities in Southern Africa, where the notion of 'parenting' can be more fluid than in many developed societies, where primary caregivers are often not biological parents, and where children may find themselves without a healthy or present caregiver for periods of time, or 'moved' to a new caregiving situation.

Above I have referred to some of the literature – including my work and that of my colleagues – highlighting the links between caregiver outcomes, such as support, health and parenting, and child health and behaviour. In my previous qualitative work, based on data and observations I argued that mutual and intergenerational bonds between older carers and the children in their care – embodying carers' commitment to see their 'new' families survive beyond their death – appeared to be one of the factors influencing their resilience and determination to survive 'against all odds' (M Casale, 2011). If protecting and providing a future for their children is, indeed, a key motivator of caregivers' decisions, outlook and behaviour, this would be important to take into consideration when thinking about support and livelihood interventions for these caregivers and their families.

What should also not be forgotten is that, in many parts of Southern Africa affected by poverty and HIV, the reality is that children often have to provide care for caregivers, family members and community members (Skovdal, 2011). While this can have detrimental effects on certain child outcomes, such as school attendance or physical health (L Cluver, et al., 2013), we must recognise this as an inevitable phenomenon in many cases, and one that may also have a positive dimension could serve as an important entry point for intervention. For example, based on research conducted in HIV-affected rural Kenya, Skovdal (2011) argues that "Although their [the children's] living arrangements and life circumstances gave them little choice but to care, a social recognition of children's capacity to provide care for fragile adults, helped the children construct an identity, which both children and adults drew on to rationalise children's continued and multiple care experiences (Skovdal, 2011)."

Moreover, we should not overlook the reality that children are resourceful and can also draw from or turn to social networks for support with hardship. For example, Skovdal and Ogutu's further research with HIV-affected and caregiving children in Kenya (Skovdal & Ogutu, 2012) showed that these children coped with hardship by mobilising and participating in friendship groups (mainly through their schools), based on sharing and reciprocal support. The children shared items such as school materials and food, and helped each other with activities such as household chores and income-generating activities. Other ways of coping included engaging income generating activities and creating positive identities around their caring roles (Skovdal & Ogutu, 2012). The authors rightly argue that developmental interventions need to recognise children's ability to access this 'peer social capital.'

I believe that an important objective for future research focus is to explore how child and caregiver social support networks and support availability are related and inter-connected. Many previous interventions aiming to improve child wellbeing by working with their caregivers have focused on their one primary caregiver, usually a biological parent, and on improving parenting. This is understandable. There is strong evidence linking better parenting to better child health and behaviour (Sheppard, 1994; Smith Fawzi et al., 2010) and some evidence showing parental social support to be a key component of successful parenting interventions and related to better child outcomes (M. Casale, et al., 2015; Hough, Brumitt, Templin, Saltz, & Mood, 2003; Richter & Naicker, 2013). But how relevant is a focus on the parenting of a primary caregiver in a Southern African context in which children may *de facto* not have one (or any) primary caregiver, or themselves be the primary carers in their home?

Clearly we need a better understanding of the more fluid and dynamic caregiving arrangements in these households. This includes the phenomenon of co-parenting, which we know is common in many African communities, as caregiving responsibilities are typically shared among various individuals in the extended family and even broader community (Richter & Naicker, 2013). But we also need to generate more knowledge on the importance of family social networks for caregiver and child health. Some of our Young Carer survey findings, described above, indicate that emotional and instrumental support deriving from caregiver support networks may have additional – and possibly greater – direct benefits for adolescent health and behaviour, over and above its effects on the primary caregiver's parenting (M. Casale, et al., 2015). It would be important to understand the mechanisms behind this, linking caregiver support networks and possibly child support. Does this show that the support caregivers receive is influencing other caregiver outcomes that we may not have measured, that in turn affect children? Are caregivers perhap providing more support to their children, beyond what we measure under 'parenting,' because of the support they receive? Or – more likely – is this an indication of some form(s) of direct interaction between members of the caregiver's support network and the children, e.g., through role modelling, advice, guidance, instrumental help? Is it a proxy of a larger and closer extended family, who may be sharing some of the parenting responsibilities? These are phenomena we need to better understand, in order to design more appropriate support interventions for caregivers and children. But these findings do point to scope for positive intervention on the psychosocial wellbeing of young adults through the broader extended family or community social network. These could include interventions that aim to boost adolescent social support and/or work with other individuals (besides the caregiver) in the young adult's social network. And this is particularly important in a context where many children have lost their biological parents, do not have a present healthy primary caregiver, or may have several different caregiving arrangements throughout their childhood.

Strengthening our knowledge on the links between caregiver and child support and networks would also be useful to be able to understand the risks and implications for children who 'lose' their adult caregiver or do not have one. Will they still be able to access the caregiver's or family's network and the benefits that derive from it? And how will this affect their own social network, assuming these can be considered as two separate entities? These are questions that can likely best be addressed through qualitative and/or longitudinal research involving network analysis.

Strengthen Links between 'Informal' and 'Formal' Support Networks and Interventions

As indicated above, there is a wealth of literature showing how the support adults receive from naturally occurring relationships and informal networks can have positive effects on their mental and physical health, as well as that of their children. These informal networks can be an important source of information exchange and support, and even a platform through which interventions may be able to better reach target populations. However, as alluded to above, how best to achieve the effects of and/or incorporate naturally occurring social relationships in interventions remains a key question and challenge. Moreover, as a result of worsening livelihood conditions, migration, and increased strain on networks in many HIV-affected communities, naturally occurring reciprocity and social networks may be breaking down and becoming less and less able to meet a large part of caregiver needs. Given the above, policymakers and practitioners need to do more to strengthen the links between informal and formal support networks.

This is another argument put forward by Skovdal and co-authors, with specific reference to children and the HIV response. The authors argue, for example, that while formal responses are central to addressing HIV, these must recognise and build on existing 'indigenous community resources' (Skovdal, et al., 2013). They explain that, in order to respond to the hardships faced by children, community volunteers and health programmes need to take into account children's roles behind the scenes, as social actors and beneficiaries of support, and understand their current support systems (Skovdal, et al., 2013; Skovdal & Ogutu, 2012). The same argument can, of course, be made for caregivers. When working in a specific context and/or with a specific caregiver population, interventionists need to gain sufficient knowledge of existing informal support mechanisms and networks, and explore ways of linking these up with formal mechanisms, as well as potentially supporting them. There may be various models for this. It could, for example, involve integrating existing informal groups within formal CBOs and NGOs or clinic support services; using informal associations as platforms for health education and psychosocial support; increasing access and uptake for interventions by working with these groups; and, where relevant, supporting these associations or networks with resources (whether monetary, a physical space to meet or assistance in setting up structures that could be easily maintained in the long term).

Another important link between formal and informal caregiving and social networks is represented by home-based carer (HBC) and community health workers. Home-based carers are possibly the most important or - in some cases - only form of contact for many caregivers who are not highly mobile and/or living in more isolated areas. HBCs, and in particular community home-based carers (CHBCs), form the foundation for extended and effective primary health care services. This is particularly reflected in the WHO primary health care model[16] and African countries' renewed commitment to revitalise the primary health care

[16] Spurred by a number of factors, including the increase and greater focus on NCDs and demographic changes in the population, the WHO spearheaded a primary health care (PHC) 'revitalisation' agenda in Africa, which culminated in the Ouagadougou declaration – where countries reinforced their commitment to a primary health care approach and strengthening of health systems to address multiple health conditions and need (Aantjes, Quinlan, & Bunders, 2014; Barry et al., 2010).

agenda (Aantjes, Quinlan, & Bunders, 2014). These place community partners, patients and family members at the centre of care provision (World Health Organisation, 2002). Community health workers are integral if the demands of individuals and health systems are to be met, in the face of an increasing need for chronic care (Aantjes, et al., 2014). However, in order to effectively carry out this role for caregivers and broader populations, HBC need to be able to assess and deal with individuals' potentially multiple co-existing health conditions and needs. This in consideration of a number of regional and global health trends, such as the increase in non-communicable diseases (NCDs), and the 'transformation' of AIDS into a chronic versus terminal disease through widespread provision of ART. The question is, once again, how best to achieve this in countries facing huge health challenges, in a context of strained health systems and inadequate resources for health. This is the situation of many of the countries in Southern Africa hardest hit by the HIV epidemic. And while there has been much debate around and recognition of the need for task-shifting when restructuring health systems, community health workers are in many cases over-burdened and not sufficiently supported with training or resources. This was shown up by a study that explored client referral patterns and practices by community care workers (CCWs) in rural South Africa (Sips et al., 2014). The authors found that community care workers had high levels of commitment but were under-resourced and even going to the extent of using their own resources to help their clients access clinics and hospitals. They called for urgent risk protection strategies to ensure sustainability of home-based care organisations and community care workers, whose success requires an enabling environment, good referral system and supply of essential commodities (Sips, et al., 2014).

Home-based care and community health workers are essential in ensuring that caregivers and their children in HIV-affected communities are provided with comprehensive primary health care for their multiple health needs, and are able to regularly access to health services and medication if they need long-term or life-long treatment (Aantjes, et al., 2014). As recently argued by various authors, this requires collaboration between formal health systems and civil society, CBOs and NGOs in community health development; however, it also requires coordination between health and social systems (Aantjes, et al., 2014; Barry et al., 2010). While there appears to be a shift in thinking and practice in this direction, considerable challenges remain. This was highlighted by a review of community home based care programmes with national primary health care revitalisation strategies in four African countries (Ethiopia, Malawi, South Africa and Zambia)(Aantjes, et al., 2014). It showed that in all four countries service provision was moving from palliative to chronic care and a diversification of care and support activities (Aantjes, et al., 2014). However, the approaches used to incorporate CHBC programmes into primary health care - including supervision, referral and contracting - differed across countries (Aantjes, et al., 2014). There were also differences in levels and mechanisms for community health and social welfare coordination, which proved to be very challenging (Aantjes, et al., 2014; Bengoa, 2013).

In sum, in order to provide comprehensive and long-term health care and support to caregivers and their families in HIV-affected Southern African communities, integration and coordination across various – formal and informal – sectors and mechanisms are crucial. This includes working with informal social networks and mechanisms and linking them to the formal (health and social) sectors, and coordinating health and social welfare services. Particularly in more remote communities and/or situations in which caregivers are not highly mobile, community home-based care is central to supporting households and connecting them to formal services. While there is clearly a shift in thinking and practice in this direction, it would appear that there is still much to be done in order to address resource and coordination challenges.

Prepare for Evolving Characteristics and Needs of Caregiver Populations in Southern Africa

Lastly, although caregiving activities continue to be borne predominantly by women, caregivers of children in Southern Africa are, inevitably, a dynamic and evolving population group, within a dynamic and evolving regional environment. The characteristics of populations providing care have changed over the past few decades, and will continue to change as a result of social, economic and demographic trends in the region. For example, HIV-related morbidity and mortality among young adults led to an increasing number of 'foster' parents, grandparents and older adults taking on primary care activities for children, as well as an increasing number of children having to take on care activities in the home. A changing HIV epidemic and the advent of widespread ART access have, however, brought about significant changes once again, and it would be important to understand the implications of these for caregiving arrangements. Young adult mortality due to HIV will of course decrease as HIV is transformed into a chronic disease through ART. These trends in the most affected Southern African countries will likely result in a shift back to a proportionately larger number of younger adults (e.g., biological parents versus grandparents) taking on caregiving responsibilities for children and the ill. However, judging from experiences in high income countries, there will be increasing chronicity and disabilities among HIV-positive individuals, linked to living a long life with HIV, opportunistic infections and treatment (Meintjes et al., 2012; Nixon, Hanass-Hancock, Whiteside, & Barnett, 2011)[17]. Moreover, the prevalence of non-communicable diseases (NCDs) is increasing at a regional and global level. It is estimated that in Sub-Saharan Africa more than two million deaths occurr due to NCDs, representing a 46% increase since 1990; these include mental and behavioural conditions and musculoskeletal diseases (Naghavi & Forouzanfar, 2013). Given the above, health risks among caregiver populations may be decreasing as a result of lower average age (due to reduced young adult mortality); however, a larger number of (mainly younger adult) biological parents and other caregivers will be on treatment for HIV, co-morbidities and other lifelong chronic disease and will be experiencing mental health conditions. There will therefore be a growing need to support biological and foster parents with comprehensive care for disabilities and multiple (mental and physical) health conditions, and to ensure that their children are receiving adequate care. This may, for example, require a different type of attention to ongoing health care and rehabilitation, for which health services and systems need to adapt. As indicated above, consideration should also be given to both the risks and positive contribution of children in this context, as they may already be taking on care and household activities for adults in their home with illness and disability, and be able to provide tangible and emotional support for healing and rehabilitation (Skovdal, 2011).

---

[17] According to the 2011 World Health Organisation World Disability report, the prevalence of disability in Southern Africa is estimated to be as around 24,5%, far higher than the world average of 15% (World Health Organisation, 2011), partly as a result of the increase in chronic diseases including HIV/AIDS.

These considerations inspired me work together with a colleague who specialises in the area of disability, to explore the relationship between disability and caregiving. Based on a review of the disability, caregiving and HIV literature, and existing disability models, we developed an exploratory model to illustrate the potential interrelationship between caregiving and disability in the context of HIV (Hanass-Hancock & Casale, 2014). We argued that co-existing experiences of disability and caregiving burden in HIV-endemic areas could lead to a vicious cycle of deteriorating wellbeing among affected households, and place additional strain on health and social security systems. We argued that research, policy and practice should aim to provide more effective synergies between rehabilitation, HIV treatment, care and support, and household livelihood interventions (Hanass-Hancock & Casale, 2014). For now this work is conceptual and exploratory, aimed at drawing attention to the 'multiple burdens' of caregiving and disability in Southern Africa, and what this could mean for individuals and systems. We hope it will spur thinking and future research on these under-explored issues. As the characteristics and needs of caregivers in Southern African communities change, so should our approaches to trying to deal with these; this requires working towards dynamic and responsive systems and interventions, able to adapt to meet these changing needs.

Conclusion

As I look back at the past decade, I am appreciative of the opportunity I have had to work directly on the ground with individual caregivers of children and their households. I am especially grateful to, and inspired by, the many caregivers who welcomed me and my research teams into their homes and openly shared their – often painful and sensitive – experiences with us. It has provided me with a particular type of insight into their world that I could never have achieved through simply analysing databases or reading the work of others. And I think this has been important in terms of making sense of and reporting findings that, ultimately, contain their stories, concerns and hopes for positive change.

But of course, with this opportunity comes responsibility. The responsibility to make these messages heard, in a way that protects participants and does not expose them to unnecessary harm (Council for International Organization of Medical Sciences (CIOMS), 2002), that best reflects the meaning and intention with which they were conveyed, and that ensures that this information reaches the relevant decision-makers in a form that allows them to understand and effectively use it. Unfortunately this is all much easier said than done, given the many challenges around research ethics and utilisation (of course, beyond the scope of this chapter). And the question of whether I have done my best in this regard is a difficult one to answer. Yes, through my own work and that of the project teams, we have travelled to present at many conferences, published a good number of academic papers (read, admittedly mainly by other academics), written up short policy briefs for specific decision-makers (which we really hope were read but will never really know), produced multimedia pieces for broader audiences, and presented findings at numerous fora with stakeholders at all levels (including NGOs, government departments, community and district authorities, international development agencies). And the Young Carers project, for example, has already influenced an impressive list of South African and international policies (SA, 2015), mainly through the networks, determination and hard work of those leading the project at a national level. But could I have done more at a personal level? I suppose one always could.

One of the things I have found difficult about being a researcher is the distance from intervention and policy change. Your role as an applied researcher is to listen, to observe, to record and to effectively convey information and – at the most - provide recommendations to those who can intervene or change policy. But you are not an interventionist and cannot attempt to directly affect change. Yet it is difficult to not be moved or affected by what you see and hear, to not want to be able to do something to help more immediately and directly. Over and above this, as researchers we often find ourselves doing a balancing act, trying to juggle the intellectual focus and skills needed for academic outputs, the practical and immediate management requirements of projects, and the type of activities and skills needed to effectively be an advocate for change. It is not always easy to get this balance right. And despite one's best intentions, success through advocacy efforts may be very slow, or invisible, or not happen at all.

I currently find myself at a junction in the journey of my own life, ready to move onto the next phase, whatever that may be. Yet my concern for and strong commitment to these populations remain. I sincerely hope that this decade of my life dedicated to better understanding vulnerability and the role of social networks in protecting caregivers of children and their families has made a useful contribution to the broader body of evidence that policymakers and interventionists can draw from. And I hope this work will be taken forward by other scholars and interventionists with similar interests and commitment, and perhaps new energy and insights. I feel as though we have come a long way with HIV- and health-related research over the past ten years. But much still remains to be done, particularly in expanding our focus to holistic health needs, and translating this knowledge into effective, targeted interventions. With specific regard to caregivers and their children living in poor Southern African communities, this will require initiatives that include: strengthening informal social networks and connecting them to formal services; providing caregivers with both instrumental and psychosocial support to face health challenges and other livelihood stressors; adapting systems and services to best meet the multiple and changing needs of caregiver populations; and better understanding the bonds between caregivers and their children and how their social networks may be connected.

REFERENCES

Aantjes, C., Quinlan, T., & Bunders, J. (2014). Integration of community home based care programmes within national primary health care revitalisation strategies in Ethiopia, Malawi, South Africa and Zambia: a comparative assessment. *Globalization and Health, 10*, 85.

Acton, G., & J., K. (2001). Interventions to reduce the burden of caregiving for an adult with dementia: A meta-analysis. *Res Nurs Health, 24*, 349-360.

Barry, S., Somanje, H., Kirigia, J., Nyoni, J., Bessauod, K., Trapsida, J., . . . Tumusiime, P. (2010). The Ouagadougou declaration on primary health care and health systems in Africa: achieving better health for Africa in the new millenium. *African Health Monitor, 12*, 10-21.

Bengoa, R. (2013). Transforming health care: an approach to system-wide implementation. *Int. J. Integr. Care, 2013*(13).

Breuer, E., Myer, L., Struthers, H., & Joska, J. (2011). HIV/AIDS and mental health research in sub-Saharan Africa: a systematic review. *African Journal of AIDS Research, 10*(2), 101-122.

Butler, L., & Nolen-Hoeksema, S. (1991). Responses to depression and their effects on the duration of depressive episodes. *Journal of Abnormal Psychology, 100*(4), 569-582.

Caprara, G., Barbaranelli, C., Pastorelli, C., Bandura, A., & Zimbardo, P. (2000). Prosocial foundations of children's academic achievement. *Psychological Science, 11*(4), 302-306.

Carlo, G., Crockett, L., Wilkinson, J., & Beal, S. (2011). The longitudinal relationship between rural adolescents' prosocial behaviors and young adults' substance use. *Journal of Youth and Adolescence, 40*(9), 1192-1202.

Casale, M. (2011). 'I am living a peaceful life with my grandchildren. Nothing else.' Stories of adversity and 'resilience' of older women caring for children in the context of HIV/AIDS and other stressors. *Ageing and Society, 31*(8), 1265-1288.

Casale, M. (2013). *The protective role of social support for the health of caregivers of children in HIV-endemic South Africa.* PhD, University of Cape Town, Cape Town.

Casale, M. (2015). The importance of family and community support for the health of HIV-affected populations in Southern Africa: What do we know and where to from here? *British Journal of Health Psychology, 20*(1), 21-35.

Casale, M., Cluver, L., Crankshaw, T., Kuo, C., Lachman, J., & Wild, L. (2015). Direct and indirect effects of caregiver social support on adolescent psychological outcomes in two South African AIDS-affected communities. *American Journal of Community Psychology, 55*(3-4), 336-346.

Casale, M., & Crankshaw, T. (In press). 'They laugh when I sing': Perceived effects of caregiver social support on child wellbeing among South African caregivers of children. *Journal of Child and Adolescent mental health.*

Casale, M., Drimie, S., Quinlan, T., & Ziervogel, G. (2009). Understanding vulnerability in southern Africa: comparative findings using a multiple-stressor approach in South Africa and Malawi. *Regional Environmental Change, 10*(2), 157-168.

Casale, M., Flicker, S., & Nixon, S. (2011). Fieldwork challenges: Lessons learned from a North-South public health research partnership. *Health Promotion Practice, 12*(50), 734-743.

Casale, M., Lane, T., Sello, L., Kuo, C., & Cluver, L. (2013). Conducting health survey research in a deep rural South African community: challenges and adaptive strategies. *Health Research Policy and Systems, 11*(14), doi:10.1186/1478-4505-1111-1114.

Casale, M., Wild, L., Cluver, L., & Kuo, C. (2014). The relationship between social support and anxiety among caregivers of children in HIV-endemic South Africa. *Psychology, Health & Medicine, 19*(4), 490-503.

Casale, M., Wild, L., Cluver, L., & Kuo, C. (2015). Social support as a protective factor for depression among women caring for children in HIV-endemic South Africa. *Journal of Behavioral Medicine, 38*(1), 17-27.

Casale, M., Wild, L., & Kuo, C. (2013). "They give us hope": HIV-positive caregivers' perspectives on the role of social support for health. *AIDS Care, 25*(10), 1203-1209.

Casale, M., Wild, L., Kuo, C., & Cluver, L. (2012, July-a). *Gender differences in social support sources and availability among caregivers of children from two HIV-endemic*

South African communities. Paper presented at the XIX International AIDS Conference, Washington DC.

Casale, M., Wild, L., Kuo, C., & Cluver, L. (2012, July-b). *The relationship between social support and self-reported health among HIV-positive and HIV-negative caregivers of children in two HIV-endemic South African communities*. Paper presented at the XIX International AIDS Conference, Washington, DC, USA.

Chazan, M. (2008). Seven 'deadly' assumptions: unravelling the implications of HIV/AIDS among grandmothers in South Africa and beyond. *Ageing & Society, 28*, 935-958.

Cluver, L., Kganakga, C., Kuo, C., & Casale, M. (2010). *Parenting, disability and HIV/AIDS: understanding impacts on children in AIDS-affected families*. Paper presented at the Symposium on Children and HIV: Family Support First - Working Together to Achieve Universal Support and Access to Treatment, Vienna, Austria.

Cluver, L., Orkin, M., Boyes, M., Sherr, L., Nikelo, J., & Makhasi, D. (2013). Pathways from parental AIDS to child psychological, educational and sexual risk: Developing an empirically-based interactive theoretical model. *Social Science & Medicine, 87*, 185-193.

Cluver, L., Orkin, M., Moshabela, M., Kuo, C., & Boyes, M. (2013). The hidden harm of home-based care: Pulmonary tuberculosis symptoms among children providing home medical care to HIV/AIDS-affected adults in South Africa. *AIDS Care, 25*(6), 748-755.

Council for International Organization of Medical Sciences (CIOMS). (2002). International Ethical Guidelines for Biomedical Research Involving Human Subjects, from http://www.cioms.ch/publications/layout_ guide2002.pdf.

Dalgard, O., Anstorp, T., Benum, K., & Sorensen, T. (1995). Social network and mental health - an intervention study. In T. Brugha (Ed.), *Social support and psychiatric disorder*. Cambridge: Cambridge: University Press.

Davies, S., Hortona, T., Williams, A., Martin, M., & Stewart, K. (2009). MOMS: formative evaluation and subsequent intervention for mothers living with HIV. *AIDS Care 21*(5), 552-560.

Davis, E., Tamayo, A., Fernandez, A., & Cresswell, K. (2012). "Because somebody cared about me. That's how it changed things": Homeless, chronically ill patients' perspectives on case management. *PLoSONE, 7*(9), 1-7.

Demmer, C. (2006). Confronting AIDS-related loss and grief: an exploratory study of professional caregivers in Kwazulu-Natal, South Africa. *AJAR, 5*(2), 97-107.

Department of Health. (2008). The national HIV and syphilis prevalence survey South Africa. Pretoria: South African Department of Health.

Dickens, A., Richards, S., Greaves, C., & Campbell, J. (2011). Interventions targeting social isolation in older people: a systematic review. *BMC Public Health, 11*, 647.

Drimie, S., & Casale, M. (2009). Multiple stressors in Southern Africa: the link between HIV/AIDS, food insecurity, poverty and children's vulnerability now and in the future. *AIDS Care, 21*(S1), 28-33.

Eisenberg, N., Fabes, R., & Spinrad, T. (2006). Prosocial development. In N. Eisenberg, W. Damon & R. Lerner (Eds.), *Handbook of child psychology: Vol. 3. Social, emotional, and personality development (6th ed.)* (pp. 646-718). Hoboken, NJ: Wiley.

Ertel, K., Glymour, M., & Berkman, L. (2010). Social networks and health: A life course perspective integrating observational and experimental evidence. *Journal of Social and Personal Relationships, 26*(1), 73-92.

Feaster, D., Brincks, A., Mitrani, V., Prado, G., Schwartz, S., & Szapocznik, J. (2011). The Efficacy of Structural Ecosystems Therapy for HIV Medication Adherence with African American Women. *Journal of Family Psychology, 24*(1), 51-59.

Futterman, D., Shea, J., Besser, M., Stafford, S., Desmond, K., Comulada, W., & Greco, E. (2010). Mamekhaya: a pilot study combining a cognitive-behavioral intervention and mentor mothers with PMTCT services in South Africa. *AIDS Care, 22*(9), 1093-1100.

Gade, C. (2012). What is *Ubuntu*? Different Interpretations among South Africans of African descent. *South African Journal of Philosophy, 31*(3), 484-503.

George, G., Govender, K., Bachoo, S., Penning, S., & Quinlan, T. (2013). Comparative economic positions of orphan, non-orphan and mixed households: Findings from round 3 of the Amajuba District Study in KwaZulu-Natal, South Africa. *Vulnerable Children and Youth Studies, DOI:10.1080/17450128.2013.772316.*

Gibbs, A., Jewkes, R., Sikweyiya, Y., & Willan, S. (2015). Reconstructing masculinity? A qualitative evaluation of the Stepping Stones and Creating Futures interventions in urban informal settlements in South Africa. *Culture, Health & Sexuality: An International Journal for Research, Intervention and Care, 17*(2), 208-222.

Gitlin, L., Burgio, D., Mahoney, D., Burns, R., Zhang, S., Schulz, R., . . . Ory, M. (2003). Effect of multicomponent interventions on caregiver burden and depression: The REACH multisite initiative at 6-month follow up. *Psychol Aging, 8*(3), 361-374.

Hanass-Hancock, J., & Casale, M. (2014). An exploratory model to illustrate the interrelationship between HIV, disability and caregiving in Southern Africa. *Journal of the Association of Nurses in AIDS Care, 25*(4), 351-363.

Harrison, A., Xaba, N., & Kunene, P. (2001). Understanding safe sex: gender narratives of HIV and pregnancy prevention by rural South African school-going youth. *Reproductive Health Matters, 9*(17), 63-71.

Herman, A., Stein, D., Seedat, S., Heeringa, S., Moomal, H., & Williams, D. (2009). The South African Stress and Health (SASH) study: 12-month and lifetime prevalence of common mental health disorders. *South African Medical Journal, 99*(5), 339-344.

Holt-Lanstad, J., Smith, T., & Layton, B. (2010). Social relationships and mortality: a meta-analysis. *Plos Medicine, 7*(e1000316), doi: 10.1371/journal.pmed.1000316.

Hough, E., Brumitt, G., Templin, T., Saltz, E., & Mood, D. (2003). A model of mother–child coping and adjustment to HIV. *Social Science & Medicine, 56*(2003), 643-655.

House, J., Umberson, D., & Landis, K. (1988). Structures and processes of social support. *Annual Review of Sociology, 14*, 293-318.

Hudson, D., Campbell-Grossman, C., & Hertzog, M. (2012). Effects of an internet intervention on mothers' psychological, parenting, and health care utilization outcomes. *Issues in Comprehensive Pediatric Nursing, 35*(3/4), 176-193.

Hughes, J., Jelsma, J., Maclean, E., Darder, M., & Tinise, X. (2004). The health-related quality of life of people living with HIV/AIDS. *Disability and Rehabilitation, 26*(6), 371-376.

Kagee, A. (2008). Symptoms of depression and anxiety among a sample of South African patients living with a chronic illness *Journal of Health Psychology 13*(4), 541-549.

Kendler, K., Myers, J., & Prescott, C. (2005). Sex differences in the relationship between social support and risk for major depression: a longitudinal study of opposite-sex twin pairs. *The American Journal Of Psychiatry, 162*(2), 250-256.

Knodel, J., Watkins, S., & VanLandingham, M. (2002). AIDS and Older Persons: An International Perspective *PSC Research Report*. Michigan: Population Studies Centre, University of Michigan.

Kühner, C. (2003). Das Gruppenprogramm "Depression Bewältigen" und seine Varianten - eine aktualisierte Metaanalyse. *Verhaltenstherapie, 13*, 254-262.

Kuo, C., Cluver, L., Casale, M., Lane, T., & Sello, L. (2011). *Parenting and Child Sexual Risk Behaviours among Children in HIV-endemic Communities in South Africa*. Paper presented at the 5th SA AIDS Conference, Durban, South Africa.

Kuo, C., & Operario, D. (2009). Caring for AIDS-orphaned children: A systematic review of studies on caregivers. *Vulnerable Children and Youth Studies, 4*(1), 1-12.

Kuo, C., & Operario, D. (2011). Health of adults caring for orphaned children in an HIV endemic community in South Africa. *AIDS Care, 23*(9), 1128-1135.

Leclerc - Madlala, S. (1999). Demonising woman in the era of AIDS: on the relationship between cultural construction of both HIV/AIDS and femininity. *Society in transaction, 32*(1), 39-46.

Lopez-Hartmann, M., Wens, J., Verhoeven, V., & Remmen, R. (2012). The effect of caregiver support interventions for informal caregivers of community-dwelling frail elderly: a systematic review. *Int J Integr Care, 12*(e133).

Mason, S., & Vazquez, D. (2007). Making Positive Changes: A Psychoeducation Group for Parents with HIV/AIDS. *Social Work With Groups, 30*(2), 27-40.

Meintjes, G., Maartens, G., Boulle, A., Conradie, F., Goemaere, E., Hefer, E., . . . Spencer, D. (2012). Guidelines for antiretroviral therapy in adults. *SAJHIVMED, 13*(3), 114-130.

Mellins, C., Ehrhardt, A., Rapkin, B., & Havens, J. (2000). Psychosocial factors associated with adaptation in HIV-infected mothers. *AIDS and Behavior, 4*(4 Health Module), 317-328.

Mukorombindo, Y., & Coetzee, J. (2013). A better life through networks and support? Vulnerable people living in a new settlement in Grahamstown. *Africanus, 43*(1), 49-64.

Naghavi, M., & Forouzanfar, M. (2013). Burden of non-communicable diseases in sub-Saharan Africa in 1990 and 2010: Global Burden of Diseases, Injuries, and Risk Factors Study 2010. *The Lancet, 381*(Special Issue S95), DOI: http://dx.doi.org/10.1016/S0140-6736(1013)61349-61345.

Nixon, S., Hanass-Hancock, J., Whiteside, A., & Barnett, T. (2011). The Increasing Chronicity of HIV in Sub-Saharan Africa: Re-thinking "HIV as a Long-Wave Event" in the Era of Widespread Access to ART. *Globalisation and Health, 7*(41), http://www.globalizationandhealth.com/ content/7/1/41.

O'Brien, K., Quinlan, T., & Ziervogel, G. (2009). Vulnerability interventions in the context of multiple stressors: lessons from the Southern Africa Vulnerability Initiative (SAVI) *Environmental Science and Policy, 12*, 23-32.

Pronyk, P., Hargreaves, J., Kim, J., Morison, L., Phetla, G., Watts, C., . . . Porter, J. (2006). Effect of a structural intervention for the prevention of intimate-partner violence and HIV in rural South Africa: a cluster randomised trial. *Lancet, 368*, 1973-1983.

Putnam, R. (1993). *Making democracy work: Civic traditions in modern Italy*. New Jersey: Princeton University Press.

Putnam, R. (2000). *Bowling Alone: The Collapse and Revival of American Community*. New York.

Reblin, M., & Uchino, B. (2008). Social and emotional support and its implication for health. *Current Opinion in Psychiatry, 21*(2), 201-205.

Reinhard, S., Given, B., N, P., & Bemis, A. (2008). Supporting Family Caregivers in Providing Care. In R. Hughes (Ed.), *Patient Safety and Quality: An Evidence-Based Handbook for Nurses.*

Richter, L., & Naicker, S. (2013). A review of published literature on supporting and strengthening child-caregiver relationships (Parenting). Arlington, VA: USAID's AIDS Support and Technical Assistance Resources, AIDSTAR-One, Task Order 1.

Rubin, K., Bukowski, W., & Parker, J. (2006). Peer interactions, relationships, and groups. In Eisenberg, N, Damon, W & Lerner, R (Eds.), *Handbook of child psychology: Vol. 3. Social, emotional, and personality development (6th ed.)* (pp. 571-645). Hoboken, NJ: Wiley.

Young Carers South Africa. (2015). 'Impact', from http://www.youngcarers.org.za/impact/

Samson, M., Lee, U., Ndlebe, A., MacQuene, K., Van Niekerk, I., Gandhi, V., . . . Abrahams, C. (2004). The social and economic impact of South Africa's Social Security System. In Economics and Finance Directorate of the Ministry of Social Development (Ed.). Cape Town, South Africa.

Sarason, B., Pierce, G., & Sarason, I. (1990). Social support: The sense of acceptance and the role of relationships. In B. R. Sarason, I. G. Sarason & G. R. Pierce (Eds.), *Social support: An interactional view* New York: Wiley.

Schatz, E. (2007). "Taking care of my own blood": Older women's relationship to their households in rural South Africa. *Scandinavian Journal of Public Health, 35*(69), 147-154.

Schraedley, P., Gotlib, I., & Hayward, C. (1999). Gender differences in correlates of depressive symptoms in adolescents. *Journal of Adolescent Health, 25*(2), 98-108.

Sheppard, M. (1994). Childcare, Social Support and Maternal Depression. *British Journal of Social Work, 24*(3), 287-310.

Sips, I., Mazanderani, A., Schneider, H., Greeff, M., Barten, F., & Moshabela, M. (2014). Community Care Workers, Poor Referral Networks and Consumption of Personal Resources in Rural South Africa. *PlosONE, DOI: 10.1371/journal.pone.0095324*

Skovdal, M. (2011). Examining the trajectories of children providing care for adults in rural Kenya: Implications for service delivery. *Children and Youth Services Review, 33*(7), 1262-1269.

Skovdal, M., Magutshwa-Zitha, S., Campbell, C., Nyamukapa, C., & Gregson, S. (2013). Children's role in the community response to HIV in Zimbabwe. *Journal of the International AIDS Society, 16*(1), 1-8.

Skovdal, M., & Ogutu, V. (2012). Coping with hardship through friendship: the importance of peer social capital among children affected by HIV in Kenya. *African Journal of AIDS Research, 11* (3), 241-250.

Smith Fawzi, M., Eustache, E., Oswald, C., Surkan, P., Louis, E., Scanlan, F., . . . Mukherjee, J. (2010). Psychosocial Functioning Among HIV-Affected Youth and Their Caregivers in Haiti: Implications for Family-Focused Service Provision in High HIV Burden Settings. *AIDS Patient Care STDS 24*(3), 147-158.

Sorenson, S., Pinquart, M., & Duberstein, P. (2002). How effective are interventions with caregivers? An updated meta-analysis. *The Gerontologist, 42*(3), 356-372.

Ssengonzi, R. (2009). The impact of HIV/AIDS on the living arrangements and well-being of elderly caregivers in rural Uganda. *AIDS Care, 21*(3), 309-314.

Stein, A., Ramchandani, P., & Murray, L. (2008). Impact of parental psychiatric disorder and physical illness. In M. Rutter, D. Bishop, D. Pine, S. Scott, J. Stevenson, E. Taylor & A. Thapar (Eds.), *Child and Adolescent Psychiatry, 5th Edition*. Oxford: Oxford Blackwell Publishing.

Szapocznik, D., Feaster, J., Mitrani, V., Prado, G., Smith, L., Robinson-Batista, C., . . . Robbins, M. (2004). Structural Ecosystems Therapy for HIV-Seropositive African American Women: Effects on Psychological Distress, Family Hassles, and Family Support. *J. Consult Clin. Psychol., 72*(2), 288-303.

Taft, A., & Brown, S. (2011). The power of social connection and support in improving health: lessons from social support interventions with childbearing women. *BMC Public Health, 11*(5), 1-11.

The Joint Learning Initiative on Children and HIV/AIDS. (2008). Synthesis Report. Learning Group 1: Strengthening Families, from http://www.ccaba.org/wp-content/uploads/JLICA-Learning-Group-1-Synthesis-Paper.pdf.

The Joint Learning Initiative on Children and HIV/AIDS. (2009). Home truths: Facing the facts on children, AIDS and poverty, from https://s3.amazonaws.com/ssrc-cdn1/crmuploads/new_publication_3/%7BD20B517E-6D54-DE11-AFAC-001CC4 77EC70%7D.pdf.

Thoits, P. (2011). Mechanisms linking social ties and support to physical and mental health. *Journal of Health and Social Behavior, 52*(2), 145-161.

Uchino, B. (2006). Social Support and Health: A Review of Physiological Processes Potentially Underlying Links to Disease Outcomes. *Journal of Behavioral Medicine, 29*(4), 377-387.

Umhlabuyalingana Local Municipality. (2011). Final draft IDP 2010/11. Retrieved 01/08/2011, 2011, from http://www.umhlabuyalingana.gov.za/ dist.php?prm1=000002.

Walen, H., & Lachman, M. (2000). Social support and strain from partner, family and friends: Costs and benefits for men and women in adulthood. *Journal of Social & Personal Relationships, 17*(1), 5-30.

World Health Organisation. (2002). Innovative care for chronic conditions: Building blocks for action: Global report. Geneva: World Health Organisation.

Yadav, S. (2010). Perceived social support, hope, and quality of life of persons living with HIV/AIDS: a case study from Nepal. *Quality of Life Research 19*(2), 157-166.

In: Caregivers
Editor: Adrienne Lloyd
ISBN: 978-1-63483-909-9

Chapter 7

COUNSELING CAREGIVERS ON HEALTH INFORMATION RESOURCES

Selim Öncel, MD
Associate professor, Division of Pediatric Infectious Diseases,
Department of Pediatrics and Child Health,
Section of Internal Medical Sciences,
Kocaeli University Faculty of Medicine,
Kocaeli, Turkey

ABSTRACT

Introduction: The internet is perceived as a prominent source of health information by parents worldwide. A survey study showed that 43% of the parents used the internet as a source of health information in the previous six months. More and more people are connecting with each other through social media (Facebook, Twitter, Freelyshout, and many others) and websites like PatientsLikeMe for being informed and supported, although informally.

The Physician's Role: The physician should be ready to face requests on reliable websites and books on general or specific health issues. In a study, 67% of patients in a community-based primary care practice agreed that clinicians should be able to recommend specific websites where they could find health information.

Health Information Media: Health information is available in print (magazines, books, newsletters) or electronic (radio, television, websites, hotlines) media. Choosing the most convenient ones will be at the caregiver"s discretion. In any case, she/he should be informed that the information is not necessarily reliable when it becomes visible to the public.

The Problem of Finding Trustworthy Information on the Internet: According to a paper by Eysenbach et al., 55 studies concluded that quality of health information was a problem on the web, 17 studies remained neutral, and seven studies came to a positive conclusion. Positive studies scored significantly lower in search ($P = 0.02$) and evaluation ($P = 0.04$) methods. In a study by Soot et al., one third of the presented information was classified by the authors as misleading or unconventional.

We have chosen Google, which is the most widely used search engine, to simulate a parent's experience in trying to find an answer on whether to have her/his child vaccinated against influenza. We searched the internet for an answer to the question "Should I make my child vaccinated against influenza?" Our findings call for the urgent need to check public-oriented healthcare information on the internet for accuracy, completeness, and consistency.

Differentiating High and Low-Quality Websites: Studies reveal that parents' inclination to believe the correctness of medical internet information and not to discuss it with the child's physician is considerably high. Taking into account this scientifically established indispensability of internet in the eyes of the modern society, it may be more prudent to increase the quality of health information on the internet, rather than trying to dissuade people from resorting to the World Wide Web for health information or decisions. Groups, such as the OMNI Advisory Group for Evaluation Criteria (omni.ac.uk) and the Collaboration for Critical Appraisal of Information on the Net (www.medcertain.org), are refining technical mechanisms by which users of the internet can easily locate quality health information in a transparent manner based on evaluative meta-information labeling and indexing. Accreditation of websites by independent certification systems, such as HONcode, may be another solution to the quality problem of the health-related websites.

INTRODUCTION

The Internet is perceived as a prominent source of health information by parents worldwide. A survey study showed that 43% of the parents used the Internet as a source of health information in the previous six months [1]. A 2013 survey by the Pew Research Center in the United States (US) found that 81% of American adults use the internet and that 59% looked online for health information in the past year [2]. Many people, especially the youngsters resort to cell phones instead of bothering to go to local library, as many individuals from the Y generation (those in the 18 to 29 year old age group) are used to practice, or even to use a desktop or laptop computer for this purpose due to the convenience and readily-availability of these hand-held devices, which have dominated our everyday life in the last several years [3]. More and more people are connecting with each other through social media (Facebook, Twitter, and many others) and websites like PatientsLikeMe for being supported and informed [4].

THE PHYSICIAN'S ROLE [5]

In this age of advanced data communication and high prevalence of technology literacy, a determined patient may be able to get access to many resources of information and gather vast amount of knowledge of interest, which may reach to amounts much more than her or his physician can look up in her/his traditional or even digital medical sources, such as books, articles, etc. If such a patient has necessary motivation and internet using skills, electronic resources in the Internet are sufficient for such a high level of personal enlightenment with medical knowledge. It may be difficult for the physician to persuade this kind of patient or caregiver about the correct and erroneous parts of this heap of knowledge. Thus the physician's skills for reading and valuation of articles, especially those having patient-reported outcomes come into prominence. Wu and coworkers propose a five-element approach for physicians when reading such a study: study design and assessment strategy, performance measurement, validity of results, context of findings, and generalizability to his own patient population [6].

Although many patients have greater access to information from a variety of sources including the Internet and other new technologies, they still do not always get the information they want or the information they gather may be incorrect. As a result of this, they are either well-informed or misinformed. Clinicians' special contributions to discussions with presumably well-informed patients should be based on competencies these patients are unlikely to have. These competencies include

- Biological basis of disease,
- Presentation patterns (symptoms and signs) of the disease,
- Understanding the process by which good science is developed and disseminated by well-trained scholars in centers of excellence,
- The process of publication in peer reviewed journals sponsored by respected professional societies,
- Critical appraisal of clinical research reports, including a well-developed appreciation of the hierarchy of strength of research designs (from large randomized controlled trials down to individual case reports) and generalizability from study patients to the person of interest,
- Appreciation of the distinction between arguments for what ought to happen based on knowledge of the mechanisms of disease, and what has been shown to actually happen in well-designed and well-conducted clinical research on patients,
- The difference between isolated observations (e.g., a case report or a single randomized trial) and coherent patterns of all relevant evidence, and
- Skepticism about information from biased sources, such as authors with financial conflicts of interest, intellectual zeal, or a wish for personal aggrandizement [7].

Efforts to make a patient or a caregiver to gain these competencies is an obvious contradiction to paternalistic medical attitude and likely to cause objections from circles supporting such an approach.

It is difficult nowadays to consider a physician who does not use the internet. An American Medical Association survey in 2009 showed that 86% of clinicians used the internet to find health information and that 29% of those accessed the internet from their office [8]. Moreover, 86% of the clinicians were found to be using smartphones in their professional activities in 2013, up from 78% in 2012 [9]. Taking into account the fact that a considerable percentage of patients come to their doctors after having searched the Internet, physicians should be prepared for internet knowledge – based questions, and approvals or objections to their recommendations by such patients [10–12]. It may be interesting, even "mandatory" for physicians to know that patients of physicians who took internet information seriously had a greater satisfaction with care as shown by Bylund and colleagues [13]. Clinicians who wish not to lag behind medical issues in the news, as it is released and not to be caught "unprepared" by patients' questions about news articles, may benefit from coverage of the top stories of the day on the web. Examples of such sites are Medical News Today and

WebMD [14, 15]. The New England Journal of Medicine offers subscribers a daily, computer-based update of medical news called Physician's First Watch [16].

Physicians should place a higher priority on patient information and education. Despite research providing evidence of the benefits of informing patients, it is readily observable that meeting patient information needs is still given a low priority by some clinicians, especially senior doctors.

Physicians should understand the patient's information needs and environment. Physicians should give their patients or the caregiver of their patients a necessary length of time tto show their level of knowledge on the issue so that the physician can decide the level of medical terminology that will be used in conversation and that errors in her/his patient's knowledge could be picked out. A well-educated person, who is using medical terminology pretty well may have low abilities to understand the implications, treatments, or the prognosis of her/his medical condition. When it comes to children, physicians should be able to estimate the general level of medical knowledge of the family and identify members of the family who take an active role in information exchange within the family. In families of high sociocultural level, the author's experience as a pediatrician and a pediatric infectious diseases specialist points to fathers as Internet "wizards," who are eager to "plunge" into the World Wide Web and take out many bits of information.

Physicians may encourage learning through reliable sources, but should not insist on patients' or the caregivers' searching health information sources, because emotional status varies among such individuals. Emotion may be a barrier to or may promote learning.

As a physician, the author's main purpose in dealing with a patient or her/his caregivers is to make them feel the comfort that, if they were treated in the most competent center on this condition, their management would be the same. In order to achieve this goal, the physician may be able to say "I have to say I don't know, but I'll go back and read about it" without the fear of being regarded as "not knowledgeable on the subject" and encourage the caregiver or the patient do her/his own readings. This will help to give the patient or her/his caregivers the impression that her/his standard of their care is not "standard," but is apt to improve and be developed by both the physician and the patient sides.

Physicians should be ready to learn from their patients or their caregivers as in the case of rapid changes in the implementation of measles vaccines in times of heavy immigration in Middle East countries, where a patient can keep track of such changes more readily from newspapers and television, let alone digital press, than can a physician with her/his sole information source of incoming official documents.

Physicians should know where to look for the most efficient and valid information. The options include colleagues, books, bibliographic databases, knowledge bases, and Internet search engines. I remember coming across a child, whose complaint was yellow sweating. Writing the symptom directly in the search box of Google revealed the probable diagnosis of chromhidrosis.

In order to avoid enlightening the patient or the parent about health information sources again and again, the given knowledge should be recorded and made visible for another health worker dealing with the patient.

HEALTH INFORMATION MEDIA

Health information resources, from which patients or caregivers of patients may benefit, are almost endless. These include magazines, books, newsletters, radio, television, websites, hotlines, and many other media.

The World Wide Web contains an extraordinary array of information on many medical matters. The websites are the most popular health information resources, because they are the ones most frequently shown by Google and most of them are freely accessible.

PatientsLikeMe is an online community built to support information exchange between patients. Their foundation story goes back to Stephen Heywood, who was diagnosed with amyotropic lateral sclerosis (Lou Gehrig's disease) at the age of 29. The Heywood family soon began searching the world over for ideas that would extend and improve Stephen Heywood's life. Inspired by Heywood's experiences, three Massachusetts Institute of Technology engineers, brothers Benjamin and James Heywood, together with their friend Jeff Cole, conceptualized and built a health data-sharing platform, which they believe, can transform the way patients manage their own conditions, change the way industry conducts research and improve patient care. The site provides customized disease-specific outcome and visualization tools to help patients understand and share information about their condition [17]. To do this, individuals can browse help topics or if they do not see the question they are looking for, they type their topic in the search bar at the top of the web page. If, after the search, they do not find what they need, they click "Submit a request." Individuals may share information about their health or they may "invite" somebody who is a site member to their "CareTeam." This new CareTeam member is selected among caregivers, doctors, therapists, spouses, and friends who help the individual manage her/his disease. Naturally, such a huge patient population provides enormous resources of scientific research. PatientsLikeMe carry out client-work, grant-funded, and internal research. Alternatively, a researcher may apply to collaborate with PatientsLikeMe or may want the help of PatientsLikeMe in referring participants from the PatientsLikeMe website [18].

The website www.uptodate.com offers two types of patient education materials: "The Basics" and "Beyond the Basics." The Basics patient education subjects are intended for patients or caregivers who want an overview and short, easy-to-read material. They were written in relatively simple language, and give insights for the major questions a patient may ask about a given condition. Beyond the Basics patient education consist of longer, more sophisticated, and more detailed articles, which are best for patients who want a more in-depth view and are relatively comfortable with medical jargon. All the patient information material in UpToDate is based on the UpToDate content for clinicians, and similar to the clinician topics. The patient topics, like physician topics, are regularly reviewed and updated. To find relevant patient information, one may type the keyword of interest in the search window and "prioritize" by patient information. Patient topics, if available, will appear at the top of the search results. It is also possible to add the words "patient information" or "patient info" to any search term to get a list of available patient information topics. The Basics patient information library is available only to authenticated users of UpToDate. Clinicians who have UpToDate access either by personal or institutional subscription are encouraged to print materials from the site for their patients. The Beyond the Basics patient information library is freely available on the web. That material can be accessed through the main search function, and through a separate patient information website. Patients who want more detailed information have the opportunity to subscribe to physician level UpToDate content for a week or month at a time [19].

MedlinePlus is the National Institutes of Health's Web site for patients and their families. Produced by the National Library of Medicine, the world's largest medical library, it provides information about diseases, conditions, and wellness issues in language lay people can understand. Patients or caregivers can use MedlinePlus to learn about the latest treatments, look up information on a drug or supplement, find out the meanings of medical words, or view medical videos or illustrations. They can also get links to the latest medical research on the topic they are searching information or find out about clinical trials on a disease or condition. MedlinePlus has extensive information from the National Institutes of Health and other trusted sources on over 950 diseases and conditions. There are directories, a medical encyclopedia and a medical dictionary, health information in Spanish, extensive information on prescription and nonprescription drugs, health information from the media, and links to thousands of clinical trials. MedlinePlus is updated daily. This site is relatively exceptional in that there is no advertising on the site and that MedlinePlus does not endorse any company or product [20].

A patient or a caregiver can find open access journals or articles on PubMed Central [21].

HealthFinder is a free service developed by the Department of Health and Human Services. It links users to reliable consumer health information megasites for health professionals. Healthfinder has resources on a wide range of health topics selected from approximately 1,400 government and non-profit organizations to bring the patient or the caregiver the best, most reliable health information on the Internet. When selecting the organizations and resources HealthFinder links to, the healthfinder.gov team reviews and considers organizations and sponsored resources that, at a minimum, meet the required quality guidelines. The team also evaluate websites based on the additional recommended guidelines [22].

Health Hotlines is a community service held by the National Library of Medicine to help the public locate health-related information. The toll-free telephone numbers in Health Hotlines were provided by the organizations and verified. Organizations listed fall into many categories including Federal, State, and local government agencies, information and referral centers, professional societies, support groups and voluntary associations. In addition to toll-free numbers, Health Hotlines also contain links to a variety of health information including AIDS, cancer, maternal and child health, aging, substance abuse, disabilities, and mental health. Health Hotlines also lists a variety of groups disseminating information on a number of specific diseases and disorders. On the other hand, The National Library of Medicine warns that it has not reviewed or evaluated the services of the organizations listed. Therefore the inclusion of an organization does not constitute a recommendation or endorsement by the Federal Government of the organization's services or views [23].

The National Cancer Institute (NCI) is the United States government's principal agency for cancer research. NCI is mandated by US law to disseminate information about cancer and cancer research and its website serves as an important means to achieving that mission. The website offers free, credible, current, comprehensive information about cancer prevention and screening, diagnosis and treatment, research across the cancer spectrum, clinical trials, and news and links to other NCI websites. The provided information is science-based, authoritative, and up-to-date. Medical experts, cancer researchers, and editors review the content before it is published to the website. The Physician Data Query (PDQ®), NCI's comprehensive cancer information database, forms the core of the information for patients and health professionals. It is regularly updated with the latest evidence-based information. The PDQ cancer information summaries are developed and maintained by the PDQ Editorial Boards. NCI also provides cancer information in Spanish. The website also provides information about NCI-supported research and NCI's grants and training programs. The site team reports on ongoing progress in cancer research through news releases, research articles, and NCI's Cancer Currents blog. The website includes links to external websites. The readers are warned that selection of external links is at NCI discretion and does not imply endorsement of external organizations or their products and services [24].

World Health Organization (WHO), European Centre for Disease Prevention and Control (ECDC), and Centers for Disease Control and Prevention (CDC) provide information on disease prevention, and health information for international travel, including recommended immunizations and prophylaxis for infectious diseases [7, 25–27].

The Food and Drug Administration (FDA) provides information on food, drugs, medical devices, radiation-emitting products, vaccines, blood and biologics, animal and veterinary products, cosmetics, and tobacco products [28].

National Institutes of Health (NIH) offers health information in sections titled as Health Info Lines, Health Services Locator, HealthCare.gov, Clinical Trials and You, Community Resources, MedlinePlus Health Info, Publication List, Science Education Resources, and Talking to Your Doctor [29].

National Library of Medicine (NLM) is the world's largest biomedical library. It maintains and makes available a vast print collection and produces electronic information resources on a wide range of topics that are searched billions of times each year by millions of people. It also supports and conducts research, development, and training in biomedical informatics and health information technology. In addition, the NLM coordinates a 6,000-member National Network of Libraries of Medicine that promotes and provides access to health information in communities across the US [30].

National Guideline Clearinghouse contains clinical practice guidelines and their summaries [31].

Created in 1984, the US Preventive Services Task Force is an independent, volunteer panel of national experts in prevention and evidence-based medicine. The Task Force works to improve the health of all US citizens by making evidence-based recommendations about clinical preventive services such as screenings, counseling services, and preventive medications. Task Force members come from the fields of preventive medicine and primary care, including internal medicine, family medicine, pediatrics, behavioral health, obstetrics and gynecology, and nursing. Their recommendations are based on a rigorous review of existing peer-reviewed evidence and are intended to help primary care clinicians and patients decide together whether a preventive service is right for a patient's needs. The Task Force assigns each recommendation a letter grade (an A, B, C, or D grade or an I statement) based on the strength of the evidence and the balance of benefits and harms of a preventive service. The recommendations apply only to people who have no signs or symptoms of the specific disease or condition under evaluation, and the recommendations address only services offered in the primary care setting or services referred by a primary care clinician [32].

American Academy of Pediatrics and American Academy of Family Physicians websites are two examples of sources of health information by professional medical specialty organizations [33, 34].

Many countries have their own official health information resources for their own citizens. In these resources, medical scientific evidence may be interpreted differently and the concluding advice may be different due to the country's own epidemiologic, cultural and financial characteristics and priorities. The National Institute for Health and Clinical Excellence (NICE) and Royal College of General Practitioners websites in the United Kingdom are two examples [35, 36].

Many universities provide good health information. Examples are Your Disease Risk by Washington University, where users can calculate their risk of cancer, diabetes, heart disease, osteoporosis, and stroke; Mayo Clinic; The University of California, Berkeley; Harvard Medical School for developed newsletter services; and Tufts University's Health and Nutrition Letter [37–41].

Medical associations like American Heart Association and Infectious Diseases Society of America have trustworthy websites that provide knowledge through their self-developed guidelines [42, 43].

For every major clinical condition such as cystic fibrosis and multiple myeloma, there exist patient advocacy organizations, which can be searched through simply Google, HealthFinder, and The Health Hotline [7].

Commercial websites like WebMD and medical research citation providing sites like PubMed, Google Scholar, and Web of Science are useful sources for the enthusiastic patient or the caregiver to get different citations for similar searches [44].

In addition to digital resources, one can get plenty of information from various books, health magazines, and medical columns of newspapers.

THE PROBLEM OF FINDING TRUSTWORTHY INFORMATION ON THE INTERNET

Finding a website containing relevant health information is often carried out by means of Internet search engines, the most popular of which, nowadays, is Google [45]. According to a paper by Eysenbach et al. 55 studies concluded that quality of health information was a problem on the web, 17 studies remained neutral, and seven studies came to appositive conclusions. Positive studies scored significantly lower in search ($P = 0.02$) and evaluation ($P = 0.04$) methods [46]. In a study by Soot et al., one third of the presented information was classified by the authors as misleading or unconventional [47].

At last but not least, we conducted a study to find out how reliable the internet is for caregivers on their decision to vaccinate their child against influenza [48]. In doing this, we aimed to find out the chances that a parent with usual Internet searching tendencies may encounter right, wrong, and irrelevant answers in her/his search in the World Wide Web. We searched the Internet by utilizing Google with "moderate filtering" (Google's default) in English and Turkish for an answer to the question "Should I make my child vaccinated against influenza?" using the keywords "influenza," "vaccine," and "children" in order to obtain and compare the global and the authors' native country's local data. Websites were grouped into eight (governmental, forum, news, interest group, non-governmental, medical professional, sponsored, and commercial) and seven (forum, news, interest group, medical professional, sponsored, commercial, and personal) categories in English and Turkish searches, respectively. The website type was determined according to the extension of the website's Internet address or "About Us" section.

Sites with "correct" answers (at least one clear statement meaning that annual influenza vaccination is recommended for all children aged 6 months–18 years), "incorrect" advice, and irrelevant content were recorded. Google searches were assessed in two ways: (1) The first ten pages of search results were taken into account because of the authors' observation that it would be unlikely for an ordinary Internet user go beyond this. (2) A separate assessment was made for the items for the first pages of the results since Internet users usually choose one of the first page results, then rephrase their search rather than exploring further results on following pages [49]. The website type and the quality of the medical content was assessed by one investigator.

As the English search revealed, 32 of the 112 websites searched had the correct answer to the question. The information contained was incorrect in 24 and not relevant to the question in 56 websites. If websites with irrelevant information were excluded, the number of sites with correct advice would rise to 64. When only the first page of the search results were taken into account, correctness and incorrectness were observed in six and four websites, respectively. There were no websites of irrelevant information on the first page of the English search results. The number of interest group websites containing accurate information (n = 12) exceeded that of sites from other categories, whereas governmental sites had the highest ratio (more than half of the websites) of correct advice. Interest group sites containing inaccurate information (n = 11) outnumbered similar sites of other categories; the same was true for the ratios of incorrectness. No sponsored site included the correct advice for the question. Five websites (three interest group and two news sites) were certified with HONcode, an accreditation given by the Health on the Net Foundation, meaning that the information in the website is ethical and reliable. Apart from HONcode, no website had a similar certification.

Out of the 103 websites searched in Turkish, 45 had the correct answer to the question. The information was incorrect in 46 and not relevant to the question in 12 websites. The number of sites with correct advice would rise to 50 with the exclusion of sites with irrelevant information. When the first page of search results were taken into account, correctness and incorrectness were observed in four and six websites, respectively. There were not any irrelevant information-containing websites on the first page of the Turkish search results either. The interest group websites (n = 22) not only outnumbered the sites from other categories for containing accurate information, but had the highest ratio (about half of the websites) of correct advice as well. On the other hand, this category had the most sites with inaccurate information (n = 17). No sponsored site in the Turkish search was found to have correct advice for the question. Sponsored sites and Internet forums had the highest ratio of information inaccuracy. None of the Turkish websites were certified with an accreditation system such as HONcode.

Our findings, together with relevant studies, call for the urgent need to check public-oriented immunization information on the Internet for accuracy, completeness, and consistency. Although a majority (88% in a study) of parents are willing to use and may be suggested to use of Internet sites by their doctors, it is our opinion that influenza and other specific vaccination information on the Internet cannot and should not be a substitute for routine care by primary care physicians [50].

In another study, taking inflammatory bowel disease as an example, it is found that few sites on this special medical topic were providing high-quality information [51].

Differentiating High and Low-Quality Websites

Believing and confirming the trueness of the information of Internet origin is another issue: Studies reveal that parents' inclination to believe the correctness of medical internet information and not to discuss it with the child's physician is considerably high. Taking into account this scientifically established indispensability of internet in the eyes of the modern society, it may be more prudent to increase the quality of health information on the internet, rather than trying to dissuade people from resorting to the World Wide Web for health information or decisions. Groups, such as the OMNI Advisory Group for Evaluation Criteria (omni.ac.uk) and the Collaboration for Critical Appraisal of Information on the Net (www.medcertain.org), are refining technical mechanisms by which users of the internet can easily locate quality health information in a transparent manner based on evaluative meta-information labeling and indexing. Accreditation of websites by independent certification systems, such as HONcode, which has been mentioned above, may be another solution to the quality problem of the health-related websites.

The Consumer and Patient Health Information Section of the Medical Library Association has a link to a list of 100 "General Health Web Sites You Can Trust.," classified as general health, women's health, men's health, parenting and kids, senior health, specific health, for health professionals, drug information resources, complementary and alternative, and other useful health sites [52].

Patients who are curious to know whether a website is of quality and reliable are advised to look up criteria developed by the Medical Library Association [53]. This tool will guide the user through a series of questions to evaluate a health information site.

The National Institutes of Health has also made recommendations for how to evaluate health information on the internet [54].

References

[1] Khoo K, Bolt P, Babl FE, Jury S, Goldman RD. Health information seeking by parents in the Internet age. *J. Paediatr. Child Health,* 2008;44(7-8):419–23.

[2] Fox S, Duggan M. Health Online 2013 [Internet]. Pew Research Center's Internet & American Life Project. Available from: http://www.pewinternet.org/2013/01/15/health-online-2013/. Accessed: April 26, 2015.

[3] Rainie L, Estabrook L, Witt E. Information Searches That Solve Problems [Internet]. Pew Research Center's Internet & American Life Project. Available from: http://www.pewinternet.org/2007/12/30/information-searches-that-solve-problems/. Accessed: April 26, 2015.

[4] Fox S, Jones S. The Social Life of Health Information [Internet]. Pew Research Center's Internet & American Life Project. Available from: http://www.pewinternet.org/2009/06/11/the-social-life-of-health-information/. Accessed: April 26, 2015.

[5] Jones RB, Hampshire AJ, Tweddle S, Moult B, Hill A. The clinician's role in meeting patient information needs: suggested learning outcomes. *Med. Educ.*, 2001;35(6):565–71.

[6] Wu AW, Bradford AN, Velanovich V, Sprangers MAG, Brundage M, Snyder C. Clinician's checklist for reading and using an article about patient-reported outcomes. *Mayo Clin. Proc.*, 2014;89(5):653–61.

[7] Guide to health information resources for patients [Internet]. Available from: http://www.uptodate.com/contents/guide-to-health-information-resources-for-patients?source = search_result&search = Guide+to+ health+information+resources+for+patients&selectedTitle = 1%7E150. Accessed: August 16, 2015.

[8] 86% of physicians use Internet to access health information - amednews.com [Internet]. Available from: http://www.amednews.com /article/20100104/business/301049966/7/. Accessed: August 16, 2015.

[9] Epocrates 2013 Mobile Trends Report - Maximizing Multi-Screen Engagement Among Clinicians [Internet]. Epecrates, Inc.; 2013. Available from: http://www.epocrates.com/oldsite/statistics/2013% 20Epocrates%20Mobile%20Trends%20Report_FINAL.pdf. Accessed: August 16, 2015.

[10] van den Bruele T, Vos HMM. Doctor, know that your patient has Googled: Internet and reason for medical consultation. *Ned. Tijdschr. Geneeskd.*, 2014;158:A8093.

[11] Sahin C, Tuncer M, Yazici O, Kafkasli A, Can U, Eryildirim B, et al. The importance of Internet usage for urologic patients. *Arch. Ital. Urol. Androl. Organo Uff Soc. Ital. Ecogr. Urol. E Nefrol. Assoc. Ric. Urol.*, 2014;86(4):261–5.

[12] McMullan M. Patients using the Internet to obtain health information: how this affects the patient-health professional relationship. *Patient Educ. Couns*, 2006;63(1-2):24–8.

[13] Bylund CL, Gueguen JA, D'Agostino TA, Li Y, Sonet E. Doctor-patient communication about cancer-related internet information. *J. Psychosoc. Oncol.*, 2010;28(2):127–42.

[14] WebMD - Better information. Better health. [Internet]. WebMD. Available from: http://www.webmd.com/default.htm. Accessed: August 17, 2015.

[15] Medical News Today [Internet]. Medical News Today. Available from: http://www.medicalnewstoday.com/. Accessed: August 17, 2015.

[16] Physician's First Watch: Medical News from NEJM Journal Watch [Internet]. Available from: http://www.jwatch.org/medical-news. Accessed: August 17, 2015.

[17] Frost JH, Massagli MP. Social uses of personal health information within PatientsLikeMe, an online patient community: what can happen when patients have access to one another's data. *J. Med. Internet. Res.*, 2008;10(3):e15.

[18] PatientsLikeMe help center [Internet]. Available from: https://support.patientslikeme.com/hc/en-us. Accessed: August 13, 2015

[19] UpToDate Subscriptions for Patients and Caregivers | UpToDate [Internet]. Available from: http://www.uptodate.com/home/uptodate-subscription-options-patients. Accessed: August 16, 2015.

[20] MedlinePlus - Health Information from the National Library of Medicine [Internet]. Available from: http://www.nlm.nih.gov /medlineplus/. Accessed: August 16, 2015.

[21] Steinbrook R. Public access to NIH-funded research. *N. Engl. J. Med.*, 2005;352(17):1739–41.
[22] healthfinder.gov - Your Source for Reliable Health Information [Internet]. Available from: https://healthfinder.gov/. Accessed: August 16, 2015.
[23] Welcome to Health Hotlines | Health Hotlines [Internet]. Available from: http://healthhotlines.nlm.nih.gov/. Accessed: August 16, 2015.
[24] Comprehensive Cancer Information [Internet]. National Cancer Institute. Available from: http://www.cancer.gov/. Accessed: August 16, 2015 Available from: http://www.cancer.gov/
[25] WHO | World Health Organization [Internet]. WHO. Available from: http://www.who.int/en/. Accessed: August 16, 2015.
[26] European Centre for Disease Prevention and Control [Internet]. Available from: http://ecdc.europa.eu/en/Pages/home.aspx. Accessed: August 16, 2015.
[27] CDC works 24/7 to protect US from health, safety and security threats. [Internet]. Centers for Disease Control and Prevention. Available from: http://www.cdc.gov/ index.htm. Accessed: August 16, 2015.
[28] US Food and Drug Administration Home Page [Internet]. Available from: http://www.fda.gov/. Accessed: August 17, 2015.
[29] Health Information - National Institutes of Health (NIH) [Internet]. Available from: http://health.nih.gov/. Accessed: August 17, 2015.
[30] National Library of Medicine - National Institutes of Health [Internet]. Available from: http://www.nlm.nih.gov/. Accessed: August 17, 2015.
[31] National Guideline Clearinghouse | Home [Internet]. Available from: http://www.guideline.gov/. Accessed: August 17, 2015.
[32] About the USPSTF - US Preventive Services Task Force [Internet]. Available from: http://www.uspreventiveservicestaskforce.org/Page /Name/about-the-uspstf. Accessed: August 17, 2015.
[33] AAP.org [Internet]. Available from: https://www.aap.org/en-us/Pages/Default.aspx. Accessed: August 17, 2015.
[34] Home | American Academy of Family Physicians [Internet]. Available from: http://www.aafp.org/home.html. Accessed: August 17, 2015.
[35] Royal College of General Practitioners | RCGP [Internet]. Available from: http://www.rcgp.org.uk/. Accessed: August 17, 2015.
[36] NICE | The National Institute for Health and Care Excellence [Internet]. Available from: https://www.nice.org.uk/. Accessed: August 17, 2015.
[37] Home | HMS [Internet]. Available from: http://hms.harvard.edu/. Accessed: August 17, 2015.
[38] UC Berkeley NewsCenter: Health & Medicine archive [Internet]. Available from: http://www.berkeley.edu/news/archives/nc_health_ med.html. Accessed: August 17, 2015.
[39] Mayo Clinic [Internet]. Available from: http://www.mayoclinic.org/. Accessed: August 17, 2015.
[40] Your Disease Risk [Internet]. Available from: http://www. yourdiseaserisk.wustl.edu/. Accessed: August 17, 2015.

[41] Tufts Health & Nutrition Letter - The Friedman School of Nutrition Science and Policy - Tufts University Health & Nutrition Letter [Internet]. Available from: http://www.nutritionletter.tufts.edu/. Accessed: August 17, 2015.
[42] American Heart Association - Building healthier lives, free of cardiovascular diseases and stroke. [Internet]. Available from: http:// www.heart.org/HEARTORG/. Accessed: August 17, 2015.
[43] IDSA : Infectious Diseases Society of America [Internet]. Available from: http://www.idsociety.org/Index.aspx. Accessed: August 17, 2015.
[44] Kulkarni AV, Aziz B, Shams I, Busse JW. Comparisons of citations in Web of Science, Scopus, and Google Scholar for articles published in general medical journals. *JAMA,* 2009;302(10):1092–6.
[45] Sim NZ, Kitteringham L, Spitz L, Pierro A, Kiely E, Drake D, et al. Information on the World Wide Web--how useful is it for parents? *J. Pediatr. Surg.,* 2007;42(2):305–12.
[46] Eysenbach G, Powell J, Kuss O, Sa E-R. Empirical studies assessing the quality of health information for consumers on the world wide web: a systematic review. *J. Am. Med. Assoc.,* 2002;287(20):2691–700.
[47] Soot LC, Moneta GL, Edwards JM. Vascular surgery and the Internet: a poor source of patient-oriented information. *J. Vasc. Surg.,* 1999;30(1): 84–91.
[48] Oncel S, Alvur M. How reliable is the Internet for caregivers on their decision to vaccinate their child against influenza? Results from googling in two languages. *Eur. J. Pediatr.,* 2013;172(3):401–4.
[49] Eysenbach G, Köhler C. How do consumers search for and appraise health information on the world wide web? Qualitative study using focus groups, usability tests, and in-depth interviews. *BMJ,* 2002;324(7337): 573–7.
[50] Tuffrey C, Finlay F. Use of the internet by parents of paediatric outpatients. *Arch. Dis. Child,* 2002;87(6):534–6.
[51] Langille M, Bernard A, Rodgers C, Hughes S, Leddin D, van Zanten SV. Systematic review of the quality of patient information on the internet regarding inflammatory bowel disease treatments. *Clin. Gastroenterol Hepatol Off Clin. Pract. J. Am. Gastroenterol. Assoc.,* 2010;8(4):322–8.
[52] CAPHIS | Top 100 Health Websites You Can Trust [Internet]. Available from: http://caphis.mlanet.org/consumer/. Accessed: August 16, 2015.
[53] Find and Evaluate Health Information on the Web | MLANET [Internet]. Available from: https://www.mlanet.org/resources/userguide.html. Accessed: August 17, 2015.
[54] Evaluating Health Information [Internet]. Available from: http://www.nlm.nih.gov/ medlineplus/evaluatinghealthinformation.html. Accessed: August 17, 2015.

Reviewed by Assoc. Prof. Zuhal GÜNDOĞDU, MD, Department of Pediatrics and Child Health Section of Internal Medical Sciences. Kocaeli University Faculty of Medicine Kocaeli, Turkey

INDEX

C

D

E

F

G

H

I

J

K

L

Q

R

S

T

U